T0095858

Let The Healing Begin

Distance Energy Healing
with Dok

Let The Healing Begin

Distance Energy Healing
with Dok

Dr. med. Christiane Wolters, M.D.

Gateways Books and Tapes
Nevada City, California

Copyright © 2018 Christiane Wolters, M.D., All Rights Reserved
Illustrations © 2018 Christiane Wolters, M.D.,
(unless otherwise attributed) All Rights Reserved
Final cover design © 2018 Gailyn Porter
Proofing: Tabatha Jones and Andrew Bishop
Editing: Andrew Bishop

No part of this publication may be reproduced or transmitted in any form
or by any means, electronic or mechanical, including photocopy, recording,
or any information storage and retrieval system now known or to be invent-
ed, without permission in writing from the copyright holders, except by a re-
viewer who wishes to quote brief passages in connection with a review written for inclusion in a magazine, newspaper, internet publication, or broadcast.

Distributed by Gateways Books and Tapes
P.O. Box 370
Nevada City, CA 95959
1-800-869-0658

www.idhhb.com
www.gatewaysbooksandtapes.com
ISBN Softcover: 978-0-89556-282-1

This book is dedicated to the ONE that lives through all of us and everything.

Table of Contents

Dear Reader

"If you have nothing to hide, full transparency is your friend."

~ E.J. Gold

Dear Reader

If you are reading this, there is a good chance you are looking for something having to do with healing, to get healthy, to "have" more energy, or you need to change your life, ease some pain that has been going on for too long. Maybe it is just a vague sense that you were meant for something more than what your life is now. Maybe you sense that the world might be falling apart and you'd like to get some things done and handled. I do not know at what stage in your life process you are, but may this book be of some help to you, no matter what level of healing is needed right now.

This is an invitation to let your healing begin and deepen. At the time of this writing, I am offering a healing space and energy work live online every Friday morning on Livestream/GorebaggTV. Everyone is welcome to be in the space. Maybe this is the time you are able to gift yourself to relax and allow healing to happen. You will find the actual link in the back of this book. It is possible however that when you are reading this, live online events are no longer happening for one reason or another.

Should that be the case, I hope and intend for this book to nonetheless be of help on your healing journey and awakening, to spark an interest in other realms and possibilities, to help become a bigger you, a healthier you, and happier you, a you that lives from a higher and deeper place, transforming into the best and greatest version of yourself. This is not a self-help program with subjects, 10 steps and x number of practices, but a general introduction to the possibility of looking past your traditional, culturally established forms of healing and taking your health and well-being into your own hands. A help to inspire you to start mastering your life, or just live it a little easier and lighter or discover your soul's purpose.

I hope to spark your interest in your healing, your evolution and in activating your full range of potential. How far you take it is up to you. It is okay to stop at any time. You are invited and called to go to the next level of what you are capable of.

May you achieve healing and feeling whole – in the deepest sense – not leaving any part out, not recoiling from or rejecting your lower or higher self, or the shadow parts of your group or nation. Find out what keeps you stuck. Allow the movement of energy through your body. Find your true core talents. Find the internal obstacles, habits or unconscious tendencies that might prevent your greatest talents from being developed and you from expressing your true greatness, living your purpose. You ARE energy and you can learn to steward your energy flow. You have thoughts and can observe how different thoughts make you feel and what they do to your energy. To enter certain vibrational spaces, you need to learn to vibrate at that level, otherwise, you don't gain access.

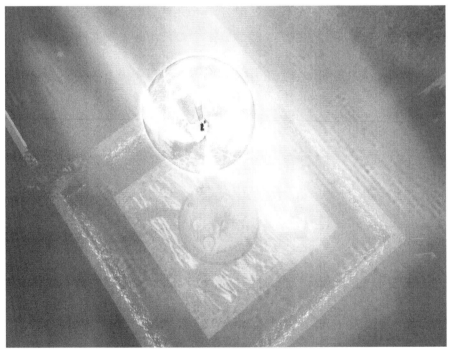

Compassionate Guardian

On this path, when you understand that nothing is excluded, that the world needs everyone, that everything is one connected big Whole, you realize: YES, may all those folks really get what they need, love in the ways they can, create beauty, laugh and be joyful. The world so needs it; creation longs for this. So it is important for you to find your inner true Self which might be buried under some fake mask you constructed to show the world. Find your talents and discover what you can do. Your happiness, power and radiant being depends on you, not something or someone outside of you. External objects and difficulties can fuel your growth, you can ask for help, but ultimately, it depends on you.

Be curious about other realms and means of perception, states of being you might have never experienced before. And no, not taking drugs – there are other means. Remember the Earth is a great healer, mindfulness is healing, real food is healing, love is healing and connection is healing.

When you think of healing and wholeness, you might have yourself in mind, your family and loved ones, or your relationships. As you get bigger, more expanded, evolved and inclusive, more and more able to see the world from someone else's perspective, when you can hold more and more seemingly contradictory viewpoints, including more and more of your SELF, you have leveled up. Your wish for healing and wholeness expands to all children, all humans and, indeed, all living creatures everywhere. There is a force of benevolence that might want to come through you. We really are all connected in this quantum universe. You might go the route of loving animals and nature and all of creation before you can approach humans. May you discover the heart of compassion and loving-kindness and Presence in the Now of your life. May you learn to pay attention to the inner voice of your essential self.

As you expand your consciousness, you may experience blissful states, you may get glimpses of the nature of the Absolute or find a meaning in your life you never dreamed was there. The saying that "ignorance is the root of all suffering" will make sense. The saying that "spirit is senior to matter" will make sense. You will understand what is meant by "the spirit that moves through all things". The saying that "all is the body of Christ" will make sense. With it comes an obligation and the energy to do what needs to be done. You may find yourself plugged in to an energy source you didn't know was there setting free your creative self in ways you could never have thought of before.

One thing one of my teachers always stressed is that the methods used to help in the awakening process are different for time, place and people. You will need to find what works for you, your type, natural inclination and talents. You will need to learn to trust what is right for

YOU, now. You will need to find the tools of transformation for you.

I do not know where you are on your healing journey. It is my hope that you will find inspiration in this little book and allow your true healing to begin and continue, as far as you wish to take it.

One word about my style of writing, or rather, my thoughts about it. I don't write too well, and admire those who are able to express themselves so much more eloquently and clearly than I am. Being a native German speaker might have something to do with it, but that is not all. Still, I write because I must, because somewhere, someone might need this, but mostly because… I heard the call.

Walk with ease and grace, dear soul, with joyful happiness in deep silence. Know there will be challenging things to face and go through to come vibrantly alive, to give your gifts in this life in a way only you can, adding to and enriching the Whole, and taking with you on your journey afterwards – a bigger soul.

Whatever the reasons are to start your healing journey, be it some deep inner pain, or an illness, you might be very surprised where it leads. The specific path we each take will be ours alone and is for each of us to discover. Each one of us has to take responsibility for finding and following our own path. Some people say: healing is not needed, you are already whole. In a way, that is true. However, the way I see it, a whole can nonetheless be broken and fragmented, parts of it entirely invisible. Part of the whole may have been traumatized and rendered non-functional. If you have an abrasion for example, you tend to it until it is healed, until the integrity of the skin is reestablished to be then again eager and able to engage that part of you in the process of your life.

The healing process includes a waking up process, a becoming conscious and integrative process. Energy work and resulting freer energy flow helps with making the body-mind more functional.

At no time does anyone ever need to wait to "be healed" to be deserving of love, care or kindness. Quite the opposite, as in the example of abrasion above. Receiving love and care is in itself healing. So is knowing what is broken so it can be mended, worked with and integrated.

In fully embracing all aspects of ourselves, light and dark, we will become open to the divine. Whatever prevents you from being a joyous being – radiating and full of energy – is in your own body-mind and psyche, a constructed "fake overlay self" to protect who you really are deep inside. In dealing with what happened to us in this life and past lives, we created a construct (defense mechanisms) that once served us, and only we can let it go. Free the energy held in place, you need it to move on. It is a path of self-discovery and honesty. A path of choosing how to be and practice new habits. Let yourself be pulled by what you love and what you are passionate about, and contribute what gifts you have. May you get bigger and stronger and may the energy flow freely through you. Let the healing begin and may you master this level and move forward, even if it is the final one of your life. May you find and trust the ground of Being itself. *For The Benefit Of All Beings Everywhere*

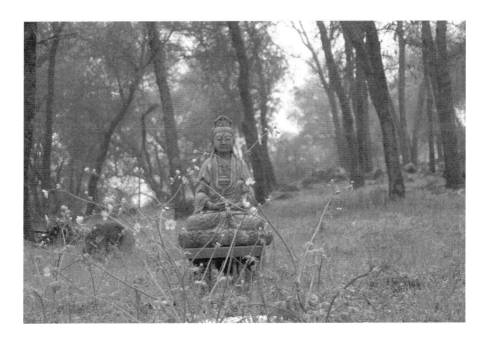

Someone asked a taxi driver in New York how to get to Carnegie Hall. The answer: "practice, practice, practice". So it is with creating new habits: repetition, repetition, repetition. Something to keep in mind.

Much gratitude to all.

Christiane, aka Dok

Enlightenment is just the beginning,
later on come other skills
....patience....
....a forgiving nature....
....extreme attention ....

~ E.J. Gold

The force of attention of the essential self is
slow and subtle. The subtle force of attention is
our only weapon against sleep.

~ E.J. Gold

Invitation To Distance Energy Healing

Healing – or, as it were, becoming whole – appears to be much needed on this Earth these days, both individually as well as collectively.

However, even though I trained in energy healing, it was not until this past Sunday, 3 days ago, May 28, 2017, that I – or something in me – got (or heard) the call. It happened in the kitchen during the preparation of lunch.

It was all laid out in front of my mind's eye. When something like that comes through, there is not much of a choice for me but to act on it, take appropriate steps and then see if it is supported, wanted and possible. (If not, I'm off the hook, so to speak.)

As it is, a live event has been added to gorebaggtv on Livestream.

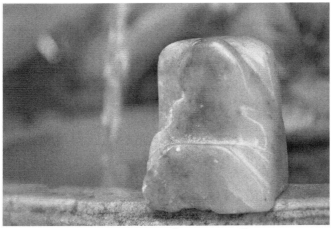

Healer Woman – Soapstone Carving

Distance Energy Healing – Fridays – on gorebaggtv on Livestream Announcement May 31, 2017

Distance Energy Healing – online via gorebaggtv
on this page – https://livestream.com/gorebaggtv
Distance Energy Work and Healing Space with Dok and Higher Vibrational Energy Beings. All are welcome. To indicate your openness for energy work: sign in, type OCD (Open-Channel-DistanceEnergyHealing) or speak "YES" in your own space.

This event is online/distance only – not on-site or hands-on

Date: Fridays – starting with orientation on June 2, 2017.

Time: 10:30 am – 11:30 am PST

What you can do to prepare for the times/space includes:

1. Create a space where you can be either lying down or sitting comfortably
2. Maybe have a mat or blanket to lie down on, pillows for knees etc., a cover or throw in case you get cool
3. If you have a Super Beacon, sit with it for a few minutes beforehand
4. Have any meaningful images or altar objects set up in the space if you wish. (This could be angelic, Mother Mary, gods and goddesses, spirit guides, teacher-images, gemstones, photos, amulets etc.)
5. Smudge the room if you can, and if it is appropriate for where you live
6. Invoke or call on your higher self or higher vibrational beings to aid or work on you. This could be saints, angel, Jesus, God
7. Cultivate an attitude or willingness for change and towards wholeness, a willingness to let go of old patterns
8. If possible, turn your phone on vibrate and leave it elsewhere

The above mentioned measures are recommended but not mandatory or necessary. You may add your own. However, it is important that you will be as physically comfortable as possible. Also here is an important point to consider: this is a shared space. Whatever care you bring to your personal space will influence the entire field. So when setting up your space, it contributes to everyone's space…we are all in the same healing space. There may be times when you don't have any extra energy to set up anything, and that is okay too, so no worries. It is good to know, however, that you are not just doing it for yourself when you bring care and attention to your own space. We are in this together.

Also, if you missed the introduction, it is available in the archives of the gorebaggtv event.

How the sessions go:

The first few minutes of the hour will be used to settle in, check mic volume (hoping for feedback from the online folks) and do some relaxation exercises.

Then the camera will be turned to an image or object or the fish tank in the space where I will be working.

A bell will sound.

The music will start – and play for about 35 minutes – the energy work happens during that time.

The entire session will be guided by higher energy and higher vibrational beings.

If you were to watch me, you could see mostly hand and arm movements. I will be moving, and removing energy blockages, balancing energy fields via energy streaming through the body and hands. Energy movements can also happen through invoked higher vibrational entities and angelic presences.

A lot of the times might simply be holding space.

If you do not wish for any energy work, no further action is required and you are welcome to simply be in the space.

At the end, the bell will sound again.

There is no charge for the energy work. There is also no guarantee you will be "chosen" – maybe simply being in the healing field is what is called for that day, maybe being open to divine energy is all that is needed.

The energy work can address all levels of the energy field.

As the higher vibrational levels get cleared, physical healing can follow. You might have heard that spirit is senior to matter… if only we truly believed that.

Anyone is welcome to attend.

It would be unlawful for me to "help" anyone who has not asked for it or does not specifically agree to it. You can indicate this by typing OCD into the chat or speaking "yes" into the space where you are. You can even specify what exactly you are asking for help with. All healings are guided. Energy will go where it is needed the most. Keep that in mind if you would like to be "worked on" or helped by higher vibrational energies and entities. Sometimes you can feel those, as for example tingling, pressure, discomfort, flashes of lifetime memories, warmth in various areas of your body, and sometimes you won't. If you don't feel anything, it does not mean there was no energy work or reconfiguration. While my perception allows me to see shapes and shades of energy and light-forms, I will deliberately not be seeing any "persons" per se. A lot of my function is holding the space of the event. If you find yourself distracted by thoughts or sensations, just whisper to yourself "yes" again to invite healing and divine intervention.

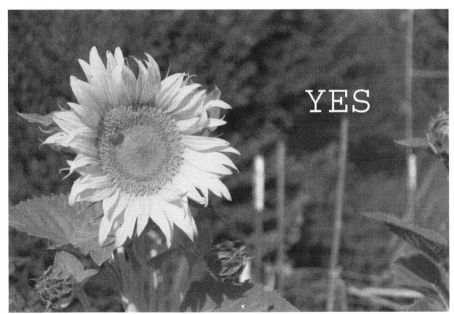

YES

Part of the energy work might in fact involve intervention of higher entities, angels and spirit guides, saints and deities. There is 100 percent trust that no effects will occur which cannot be handled by the recipient.

In a way, it is similar to the healing circles already happening in the Prosperity Ashram, or LRS healing readings or prayers.

After the music stops, especially if you were very relaxed, please be gentle with yourself. Give yourself at least a few minutes or longer, as long as you need, before getting up. **After getting up, drinking a glass of water would be a good idea**. Driving might not be a good idea right away.

Keeping a diary over the week, noting effects can also be very helpful. There is a Prosperity Path Forum where you can share experiences as well as add comments when I post the link to the notes on Facebook. At this time, there is no plan to create a group, but, depending on how things go, there might be one in the future, if the need arises. Also remember: you can help your body re-adjust towards healing/wholeness simply by not ingesting any crappy, pesticide-containing fake "foods" or beverages.

What makes me think I can do this?

First off, anyone fundamentally and basically can transmit energy deliberately. It requires intention, clarity and willingness. We Westerners, or maybe people in general, are just not taught about this – but as many mothers will know, placing her hands on an "owie" of a little one can just take the pain away. Intuitively, we still know.

The main reason is: I got a mandate and accepted the obligation. I trust that this is for the benefit of those attending, all beings everywhere and in the highest purpose of the One, God, the Absolute.

On the human level, there are some influences and more traditional "credentials" that I will list here:

- First, my own journey towards healing and wholeness leading to this expression of who I was meant to be and what I am to do at this point in the grand scheme of things.

- 20 years in the medical field working as a pediatrician and in the NICU (neonatal intensive care unit).

- Being a student of Tom Brown Jr. in a number of philosophy classes back in the early 1990's and being introduced into the world of spirit, energy, non-physical beings and the method of healing that is used in the system he taught. In fact, through all other trainings, I have often gotten back to what I learned there.

- Graduate of the four-year Brennan Healing Science program of the Barbara Brennan School of Healing (2000)

- Graduate of the two-year Hakomi training (2003)

- Maintaining an Energy Healing Practice for two years prior to moving to California in 2003

- There were other influences, of course, like Reiki, growing up in a country where "alternative" healing methods were commonplace, and I won't mention other, parallel lifetimes, but okay, I did meet one of my healer shaman selves during one of the PUP levels in <u>Beacon Training level 1</u>.

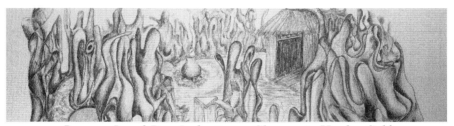

Beacon Level Pup Induction – Shamanic Healer Self

A drawing of the world of a shaman healer, jungle like on the outside, but replete with teleport and a "hut" where healings happened. They travel in transparent gliding spheres, not shown.

Why am I offering this now? Because I got the call 3 days ago, on Sunday, May 28, 2017. It is a matter of service and I would not have gotten the call if I were not able to do it or if it were not needed. So the next day I gave the music to Oz, our sound engineer, who agreed to put it together, and talked to my teacher, who supports it ("I thought you should be doing this all along" – oh well). The world seems to need it. We'll see what happens.

What about the healing relationship?

Yes, that is very important, in fact, for some phases and parts of healing, being in a therapeutic relationship might very well be needed. One such relationship is that between a caring, competent healer and the client. I fully encourage you to seek such a person or helper if called to do so. However, what I am inviting you to and am offering is not that type of one-on-one relationship.

The invitation is to receive energy work, yes, and to spend time in high vibrational fields. At the same time, it is your active participation that is required, mostly in the form of showing up, saying "yes" and to trust that healing energies will be flowing. It works a little differently than traditional models. I am holding the space, and am doing some of the energy work. Guides and higher vibrational beings do most of it. You are the one who sets up your own space, you are the one starting to care for your physical, mental, emotional and spiritual body and being. The first step in healing is establishing a relationship to all parts of yourself, discover all parts of yourself and take care of yourself.

Having said that, I add that, yes, there is a connection between the healer and healee, the one receiving energy work. As Tom Brown Jr. told us many years ago, sometimes after energy work, you will be feeling connected to someone without really knowing why.

My offering is one of service, of energy work and holding space. Going by the feedback so far, it has been beneficial for a number of people.

In any case, it is what is possible for me to do at this time and it is what I was called to do.

Regardless, start living from a connected place/space. Connect with who you are. Be kind to yourself. Love heals.

Truth be told, I am loving the DEH spaces. The times and spaces during the Distance Energy Healing have included some very high vibrational spaces. They have, among other things, been nourishing, beautiful, amazing, felt limitless and vast. It is my hope and wish that you can allow yourself to relax and "go there", to care for yourself enough to take the time for yourself and healing. If you are in a place where you can hear the transmission, it is safe enough. Allow the cells of your body, and you, to feel safe. You can learn to trust your intuition and the visions you will sooner or later be receiving, and follow your path.

The weekly time set aside for your healing could become a ritual and stepping stone on the path to the next higher level of your life. It also is part of your energy body maintenance practice.

Can you tell others about this? Yes, you may. Anyone can be in the space. All are welcome. Let them know to indicate openness for energy work, by signing into the chat and typing OCD (Open-Channel-DistanceEnergyHealing) or to say "YES" in their own space. Is there any part of the world where more wholly-healed individuals and environments would not be beneficial? It would be good if everyone participating would read this information.

You remain, at all times, responsible for yourself, and just as with the PUP inductions in the Beacon Training, nothing can happen without your consent.

The distance energy work and the healing spaces which you participate in are to support your health and well-being on the path you are on, providing a safe space for healing on many levels. Sometimes an energy influx is all the body needs to re-align and self-heal; something bodies have a natural tendency to do. Today, more than any other time in our life, we are called to go all the way and allow transformation and healing to happen from within. Sometimes all we need is a safe space and a little energetic jump-start for the ball to get rolling.

Any increased sense of wholeness will reverberate with any living creatures you come in contact with. Please note that "I" am not doing any healing. I agreed to be a vessel through which energy can flow – as guided by divine higher self/forces. If your Self gives permission for energy to flow through blockages and stuck energy structures of the energy field, things may start moving in ways they did not before. Hence, self-observation and keeping a journal are recommended.

Many blessings on your path. May you walk with ease and grace.

Christiane Wolters, M.D.

The Call

For a few years prior to offering the online event – Distance Energy Healing – I was wondering why it was that I was not doing any kind of healing work, at least, nothing outwardly recognizable as such, and had no interest in taking any steps in that direction? After all, I trained in that field. A couple of decades ago, healing work is what came to me when asking myself what I wanted to be and do. Actually, not so much being a healer, but a benevolent healing force in this world, for animals and humans alike – just generally a healing force. For what I mean by Healing, please check the chapter on "What Does Healing Mean?"

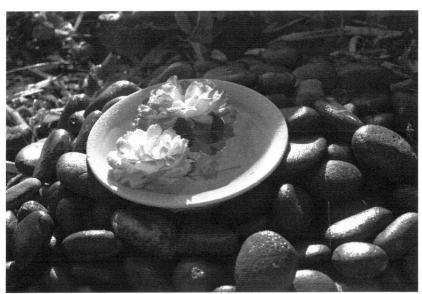

Offering

My life choices already reflected my basic disposition to service and earlier this year there was no indication that I would be doing anything other than what I was doing. My plate was very full, so full that many things were not getting done. In addition, in recent years there were times I was in so much pain physically that it was getting difficult to do some everyday chores. I even started investigating CBD oil or becoming a grower to be able to juice this god-given holy herb. Alas, it is still not legal like sage or oregano is. I decided to get back to some baseline health maintenance using the staples of diet and exercise, rest and earthing. Juicing helped tremendously. In any case, I was happy with the results.

Even with the discussion of alternative healing centers at my place of work, the loss of affordable healthcare in the USA, and the general state of the world, the environment and all the living creatures (who I dearly love), I still felt no drive towards doing healing work.

It was quite surprising then when on Sunday morning on May 28, 2017, during the preparation of lunch, the call came. It is difficult to describe "the call", but I knew, I just "heard" it… the action steps and form were all presented to my inner eyes. The inner being in me knew. It felt like a download. It might have been part of a larger shift.

A couple of weeks later, my human self explained it like this: the reserves got called in. Looking at the world as a game of good vs evil, who appears to be winning? What is needed? Exactly, so, a certain level of the reserves were called in. It's time, it's now, come. Time for humans to heal, that is, to wake up and take responsibility.

In any case, what followed seemed effortless. I took the steps and started doing Distance Energy Healing, simultaneously writing this little book to get out there while there still is time to attend them live, and so far, I am loving both.

When you get a download like that, or, when the reserves are called in, it does not matter if you think you can do the job, whether or not you feel worthy or if you conclude you can't do a job as well as someone else. (Though it is true.) None of that even crossed my mind; I am only mentioning it here because later those thoughts briefly entered into my head. All that does not matter when you – your higher self – are called to do a job. And that I am doing as best I can.

You are invited to read through these former blog posts/chapters and join in the online Healing Space, live or in the archives.

The Distance Energy Healing events are happening – until they don't. They are transmitted on Livestream – gorebaggtv. You are invited to attend live, or use the archives, as long as they are available, or just tune in.

https://livestream.com/gorebaggtv/DistanceEnergyHealing

Maybe it is time for you to let the healing begin.

Time to move to the next level.

Blessed be all things and beings.

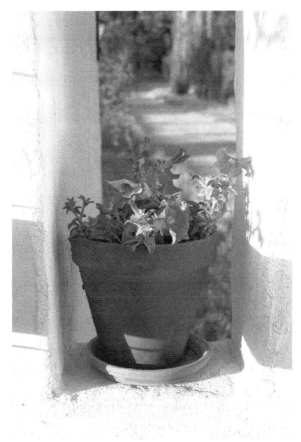

Another World Beyond

"The choice of gracefully performing your essence task or going through life kicking and screaming and bitching and griping about how unfair it all is, is again, entirely up to you."

~ E.J. Gold

"Do it now. The future is promised to no one."

~ Wayne Dyer

What Can I do

To Participate In The Healings?

The first thing is – you show up, either live online, or be there with the help of the archives. Time and space are not linear.

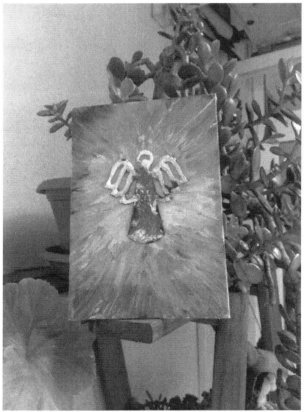

CQR Quantum Healing Angel

Image courtesy of Carmen S.

The healing space is a shared space. We, the participants, are literally creating it together and are in it together. It is not uncommon for experiences to be shared, even though one would not necessarily know it without actual sharing afterwards, at some point. Sometimes there is a common thread several participants have as important issues that week.

When you bring care, attention and a sense of reverence to the space, it contributes to the states attained and the power of the process. The deeper each one is able to relax and trust the process, the more it helps others to go there. It is simply that connected – quantum connected.

Any work you do is work for all of us, but I digress.

You can hold the intention of healing, align with the highest vibration.

You can be curious.

You can bring an open mind and heart to experience something new.

You can set up an altar or have a little ritual you do when joining the space.

You can make sure you are physically as comfortable as possible.

You can be willing to breathe consciously and relax.

You can be willing to play with having a different thought and see how that changes how you feel.

You can ask for help aloud in your space, you can define what you need help with or what you long for most.

You can call on your guides, angels or invoke your higher self.

You can suspend judgment for the time and allow benevolence, awareness, relaxation and guidance come through for you.

You can pay attention during the week to any differences you don't really have an explanation for. For example: you might be used to eating a certain food a lot, but now, you notice you don't really want it that much… and in order to act on that, as in not eat as much, you'd have to notice it first. The more clear you get, the better for everyone.

You can be willing and open to some changes in your life, changes in what you do to your body and mind, changes to the space you are in, changes in ways you speak or do some things.

You can do simple things like place your hand on your body, especially your heart, and thank it for doing its job. In the case of your heart, thank it for still beating after all it has been through and after all it has felt. You can tell it and feel the love for it. You can notice what it and you feel when you do that. The same is true for any body part: your back for carrying so much, your hands for doing and holding and... the list goes on and on. Every part of you has been doing the best it can in your life, no matter what happened.

You can follow the guidance you get. You can seek medical help or nutritional help or body work help.

You can start doing art or music.

You can listen.

You can just be there.

You can allow yourself to be held through the energy.

You can be willing to allow feelings to be there that might come up.

You can become more aware and witness what is happening.

You can cultivate the notion that we are not set in stone and rigid, but beings of energy and light and that with consciousness and intention, you can manifest differently.

If you feel this could benefit someone you know, you can tell them about it.

This list could go on for a while, and I may add to it at some point. It should give you enough of an idea about what you can do to participate in the healing.

The main points are: you show up, sit or lie down comfortably, you say "yes", you don't attach to thoughts, feelings or sensation, but are present and allow the higher energies or divine presence to transform you. You are gentle with yourself afterwards and have a glass of water.

"Suffering is the price one pays for ignorance and freedom is the reward for courage. Take your choice, it's your choice to make."

~ E.J. Gold

"Conflict cannot survive without your participation."

~ Wayne Dyer

Your Healing Altar – Do You Need One?

While the healing music is playing during the GorebaggTV healing event, the camera is generally focused on the altar space and the items on it: a small soapstone carving of a healer woman, a CQR Quantum Healing Angel, a Quan Yin statue with a Silver amulet representing groups and group genius as taught in Matrixworks, a Himalayan salt lamp light, a clear quartz crystal, a Tibetan singing bowl and a couple of other items.

Oh man, does anyone really need an altar for healing to happen?

No, not really.

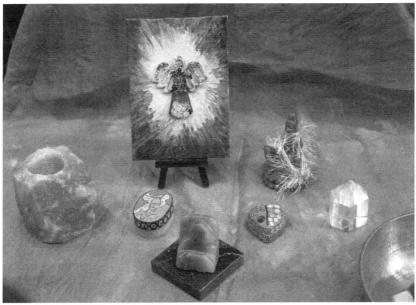

Distance Energy Healing Altar

Let us consider, however, the function of an altar space.

Commonly, "altars" are places that mark a space as not common to everyday life, but indicate that something is happening or practiced here that is of a spiritual, non-everyday, non-ordinary nature. You can find such special places, altars, in all corners and cultures of the world. Many people have an altar type place in their homes – their sacred place, a place of stillness for letting go of the mundane to connect the deeper part of themselves and with higher vibrations, spaces, angels, spirit guides or deities.

Altar objects are items of special spiritual significance to the person involved. If you have an altar, you most likely have several items on it. Some items, like prayer beads, especially blessed ones, can definitely acquire the status of sacred.

Depending on religious practices, beliefs and insights or tendencies, different people may choose different objects to place on the altar. These altar objects usually hold a very special meaning and are held in highest regard. They may be useful in accessing altered states of consciousness and often are imbued with special energy. They can function as connecting devices to a deity, spiritual school, group, space and more.

Altars do not have to be expensive to function or convey a sense of the sacred. Basically, anything you set up for the purpose can function as an altar.

Why would one want such an altar space?

"One" would want it to help facilitate non-ordinary states of awareness or awakening, to have a place to pray or sit in stillness. A place where non-ordinary states of consciousness are invoked and the ordinary worldly concerns are left behind. It is where we intend to access higher spaces, the divine, the sacred, unity or higher guidance. It can be used as a centering device, for invocation, to pray, to slow down and access a space of going with the flow, an open heart and compassion.

One of the most important conditions for accessing altered states of consciousness is the switching from beta brain predominance to other brain-wave states. This can be induced with the help of sounds, scents, moods, meditation, relaxation techniques and through one of the most potent tools I have encountered: the Beacon and the SuperBeacon.

Some altars are special purpose altars, such as Labyrinth Readers' altars.

While the connection between reader and voyager is non-physical and requires nothing other than the essential tools which are natural to all beings, attention, presence and will – our experience as readers is that a properly equipped altar dramatically assists in the process of reading.

Over time, the reading space, or generally, any altar space that is used as such, gets charged, and merely sitting down can trigger the body to change states.

If you have ever gone into and sat in one of the old churches in Europe, you can feel the space difference. This difference is not merely due to the building itself, but also the many many people, for over a thousand years, have come here for contact with the higher.

Sitting there in one of those churches, you can feel the connection to many thousands of people through the space. You can train your body to relax and go into certain spaces just by gazing upon the items of an altar space.

The healing room I used to practice in had a lot of items in it that were meaningful to me. These days, the physical space available to me personally is very very small, so the items I use are the handful that are most meaningful and imbued with energy. The items have a history and connection to various groups and higher vibrational spaces.

Keeping them around reminds me of those spaces, the higher beings and energies, and it becomes easier to slow down and get connected. The objects on my little healing table-altar are related to and resonant with the basic idea of healing, helping, awakening, transformation and service, as well as divine play and joy.

Seeing them, touching them, deliberately placing them onto the altar table each week slows me down and facilitates the best state of being for the healing space. There is a sense of gratitude. Having altar items in the space can invoke the spaces, times, groups and teachings and teachers they were a part of originally. It invokes the guides and higher beings, it welcomes help and trusts that it will be given in the form needed. It invokes the guides and higher beings, it welcomes help and trusts that it will be given in the form needed.

What this does to the body-mind is this: it relaxes it and makes it receptive – receptive to guidance and energy flow. This is combined with the intention and all this facilitates the opening of the healing space. Once the energies flow, healing and integration happen.

An altar is an aid, a reminding factor, a connector to spaces and beings and vibrational energies. It can function as a trigger point to another reality.

The act of deliberately placing the items on an altar can have the effect of a tea ceremony.

It can work that way for you.

And now, back to my original answer. No, you don't need a healing altar. But it may help you with the process.

E.J. Gold said the same about the SuperBeacon: it is an aid… and ultimately you won't need it anymore. Until then, keep using the SuperBeacon to allow the non-beta states to happen and to connect with Parallel Universe Personae. Altars are like that, too – they help.

Tom Brown Jr. said to us something like that. There could be a time when you don't have those items (in the shamanic native American tradition, these would be things like pipe, smudging, sweat lodge, bones, rocks, drums, etc) available to access this relaxed state, inner vision and the spirit world. So he taught the breath-to-heart meditation that your body learns to see as a trigger to go into a certain state of altered consciousness.

There will be a "time" after we leave this earthly plane, where even that is no longer available to us. Having trained your mind not to panic will help.

We can bring awareness to the altar objects and their placement with that same goal in mind: openness, receptivity, willingness to connect with what we call the divine, spirit or highest vibration. Use the tools you have and that work for you.

In that state, we don't just hear from others or know mentally that we are all connected, we know it – because we perceive it.

The Healing Space is a shared space, a vessel, or, as E.J. called it, a frame. And we are in the frame together, and we create it together. What you do and how you approach it, matters to all of us.

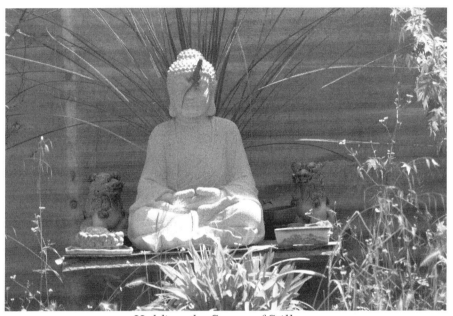

Holding the Space of Stillness

"Be in the present, it'll make a nice change."

~ E.J. Gold

"The Great Work consists in transforming a helpless other-directed puppet into an inner-directed unified being that understands its place in the scheme of things."

~ E.J. Gold

CQR Quantum Healing Angels

One of the objects on the altar set up for the distance healing spaces on gorebaggtv is a CQR Quantum Healing Angel. Why?

Because I am specifically calling on higher entities, angelic forces and divine energies to help us. Below you find more specific reasons why they are called CQR Quantum Healing Angels, and why they are the colors they are.

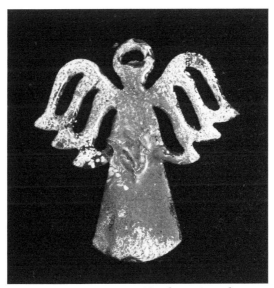

CQR Quantum Healing Angel

Why quantum? Because that is how it works in quantum mechanics: spooky action at a distance. This is spooky healing at a distance. Only it is not spooky, it just is that we really are connected. The crystal quantum radio circuit embedded in the angels connects with that quantum space specifically. **These functional crystal radio circuits – **powered by waves emanating from the stars and the explosive force of the Big Bang at the moment of Creation – **work on a very subtle level.**

Why angel? Because it signifies and connects with higher vibrational (not usually physical) entities or energies to aid or guide us on our earthly journey. Usually the word angel comes with a positive connotation, whereas "spirits" can bring up other feelings. Higher vibrational entities or energies, spirit guides, angels – they all can be called upon. I am calling on healing angels, higher beings and consciousness to help us with health, well-being and awakening.

Why are angels shown with wings? To indicate they are beings that can fly – as in… move through the air, teleport. Do they really need wings for that, given they don't have physical bodies and this is in quantum space? No. Ancient alien theorists even go so far as to say that angels are really otherworldly beings, aliens, who visit us, and use spaceships to fly. In any case, showing a figure with wings is an immediate reminder that we are not dealing with a mere mortal human.

Why healing? This is made for a healing event, hence healing angel. Many traditions talk about entities who come to help humans. The archangel Raphael (Hebrew: "It is God who heals") is one of them. He is considered the healing angel in the Christian religion. What makes this CQR angel a healing angel? The colors.

Why these colors? The healing angel Raphael is associated with the color green. Modern medicine determined that certain colors have a soothing and relaxing effect on humans – greens and blues. Our body-minds are still very connected and receptive to the sky, the seas, and the green color of trees and plants – and respond with relaxation. Some colors are more neutral, and some are stimulating and invigorating – sometimes to the point of eliciting a fight or flight disposition. Myself, I have always preferred blues and greens.

This does not mean that in color therapy, for example, you would not choose or need other colors.

Since, in a healing space, relaxation is more effective, the CQR angels were made with those colors – mostly greens with a touch of blue, plus white to signify light and purity of intention, and some with a sprinkle of purple.

Charging objects. Some of the objects of my healing altar were charged during their creation, and from being in many higher spaces already.

The CQR Quantum Healing Angel is charged from how and where it is made. Being in the healing spaces, it will continue to charge and eventually become a highly psychometric artifact.

Quantum Healing Angels can become very special altar objects. You can do this with any of your chosen altar objects.

I hope this explains my choice to include a CQR Quantum Healing Angel.

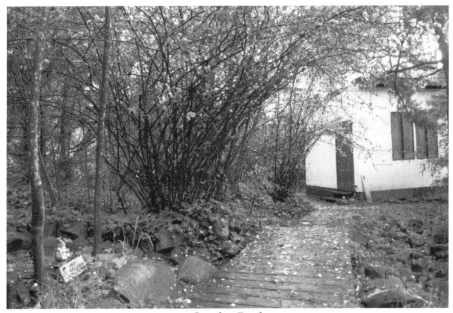

On the Path

"There's nothing like experience to teach wisdom."

~ E.J. Gold

How Does Distance Energy Healing Work?

Let us start from the point that you have accepted that energy exists, that humans have an energy field and in fact, are entirely made of energy. We already know that energy can be charged, changed, be made to flow using hands of light or healing touch. That still does not explain why it works at a distance.

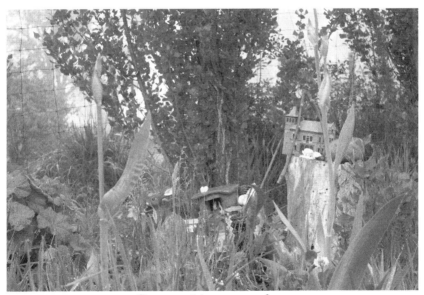

Communities everywhere

It works because that is how the universe is made. There is evidence of long distance shamanic healing "entity" or evil spirit dispelling, and maybe some would say all I am doing is casting out evil spirits; my mother would say something like the saints and angels helped us or God helped us; others say the spirit guides helped. These days a lot of healers would say Distance Energy Healing works because there is a unified whole of all that is, or it works because of quantum physics, because of non-locality, because the universe is structured in units enfolded in ever-increasing complexities, because it is a hologram, because this means we are all connected and you partake in the same healing space. It works because, energy and consciousness work together. It works because of intention and belief, it works because it is part of evolution.

Everything vibrates and you can tune into that vibration, be it high or low. Prayer has been shown to have long-distance effect.

Fundamentally, we don't really know at this time how it works, at least not that it is explainable to everyone. What I can say is this: after the first few of our distance healings, there was positive feedback about the effectiveness. You could say: those people participated, had intentions for themselves and that is what made it work. The healing space was simply a vessel, a container, an inspiration for it.

On some level, all of it is true. Miracles do happen. All of these have in common the component of intention, trust, openness, belief and focus. Yes, let us hold the intention for deep healing and transformation.

Let's remind ourselves that all that is manifest is in reality energy, swirling patterns of energy of various frequencies. We are some form of energy – or energy waves, more specifically. Everything is connected to everything else. Everything vibrates at certain frequencies. Various states have a certain frequency that you can resonate with. Matter is the most dense, solidified or slowed down energy, but nonetheless is still, at the atomic level, vibrating energy waves. Every particle vibrates at one or the other frequency. It is also always both like a particle and like a wave, with potential to go into various particle shapes, depending on the observer. This is important.

A lot of folks say that the reason distance energy works has to do with quantum mechanics, though how exactly it works still eludes even the latest science. It would take me 20 years to study and try to understand the mathematics of it, if I even could, which is doubtful.

Here is a quote by Niels Bohr: *"If quantum mechanics hasn't profoundly shocked you, you haven't understood it yet. Everything we call real is made of things that cannot be regarded as real."*

Energy waves are always meeting and getting entangled with each other.

One could say that there is spirit that moves through all things, a force that can take or inspire various forms. We, in fact, are swirling patterns of light in infinite extension, which consciousness has focused into being as us, incarnate here, and it causes "healing".

A mysterious life force that allows us to do things in life has been called by various names: prana, chi, ki, Great Spirit.

Not just from the spiritual traditions are we told that we and everything are connected. Quantum physics is now telling us the same thing. All of the entire universe was once condensed into something tiny and for better or worse, it is still connected. Some force flows through it all and binds it all together. It still is all ONE. It is all still entangled. There are things our minds still can't quite grasp: spooky action at a distance, dark matter, instant telepathy, morphogenic fields. Science is inching up to it, but the final evidence may actually be found in direct knowing.

There are forces in nature that science is only beginning to understand. Various studies have by now been done looking into effects of praying. What physicists are saying to us presently is that there is a realm of reality which goes beyond the physical, where we can influence each other from a distance. Out of the void arises what is.

Eugene Wigner, a theoretical physicist and mathematician, emphasized that it was not possible to formulate the laws of quantum mechanics in a fully consistent way without reference to consciousness.

In quantum physics, subatomic particles far apart respond simultaneously, at a distance that would be many many thousands of light years away. Spooky action at a distance. Even time and events in time are not fixed. Something still undefined binds us all together, beyond time and space, through other dimensions than just the three we commonly know.

All things are energy and in addition to the part that we perceive with our usual ordinary senses, we can also learn to see the more subtle energy forms directly, as well as the energy field associated with each physical thing or living being. Some call the energy fields associated with living creatures the aura.

Humans have an energy field associated with them, extending 3-15 feet out, and including through space and also occupying the body. It is an organizing bio-energetic field of the etheric body. This energy body has openings, vortexes, which metabolize and guide energy flow through the entire system. We generally refer to those spinning vortices as chakras. In addition, all organs are associated with auric fields. There is a blueprint for all organs, which then form according to the blueprint.

Modern science is beginning to be able to measure some of the energy fields associated with bodies, like the electromagnetic energy field of the heart.

Disease, or rather, non-well-being of the physical, has associated energy and/or auric changes in the human energy field. In energy work, this gets addressed. Sometimes it is simply charging and balancing the energy field that is needed, sometimes specific energy blocks or densities get addressed. Generally, healing energy is automatically going where it is needed.

High intensity, focus, clarity, purity, high concentration and attention are all factors that make energy work more effective. So is compassion and genuine caring.

The entire universe consists of energy. The Earth is a giant ball of energy. Energy is all around us. In some traditions it is called chi, prana, orgone, universal energy, life force. In some Eastern medical systems, the paths and nodes of the main energy flow and convergences in the body are known and are called meridians. Humans have chakras that draw in and channel energy flow. Ancients very well might have known the energy vortexes of the earth and used them with pyramids to provide electricity.

The expression of energy is guided by consciousness and intention, in humans starting at the essence or soul level. There is a blueprint for each of us. Some call this meta-programming. Depending on each person's soul, earthly origin and upbringing, energy flow gets channeled a certain way, but often, though trauma, cultural beliefs and patterning from infancy, energy gets blocked, gets stuck, is prevented from flowing. This leads to sub-optimal structure development, performance and functioning. The more freely the energy can flow, the more vibrant, clear and powerful the being.

The source of every problem can be linked to our subconscious mind, which is our cellular memories. That is where our habits and all beliefs reside, conscious or unconscious. They then hold energy forms and certain flow patterns in place, not allowing for the energy to flow freely, or only allowing for the energy to flow in certain ways. This can, over time, lead to the malfunctioning of associated physical parts of the individual.

Someone doing energy work has usually developed a way to perceive the energy bodies associated with the physical body and is able to channel energy into the field and more specifically to the stuck, dense areas. The development of high sense perception is something that can be learned by anyone, though as, for example, with music, some may have a higher talent for it than others.

Not all individual disease starts in the higher level of the field. Sometimes the polluted environment, both physical and psycho-emotional, can lead to change in the physical, leading to malfunction of affected tissues and organs. However, the individual's insistence to continue adding toxic substances to their body and energy field do often lie in fixed beliefs and energy structures of that individual.

In some shamanic systems, a lot of western "mental illness" is caused by a spirit being trying to merge with a human to channel messages from other dimensions.

One of the main ingredients of healing is connection. For you and I this means one's connection to the body and the connection of the parts of the body to each other to become a whole organism. Also, connection to the Earth and nature and all that is, and realizing we are not separate from it. There is connection to each other, and in the case of working with a healer, a connection to them. You are also connected to all of humanity, and may pick up "vibes" or know what is going on with people dear to you or those whose energy you are in resonance with. Then there is connection to one's soul/essence and the divine. All those play a role in the expression of wholeness and well-being.

The essence/soul is informed by the body-mind and vice-versa. During a lifetime, they do become intimately connected and form a whole. The soul, or essential self, appears to seek a compatible physical self in each new incarnation. In fact, one could say that the soul shapes and forms the body. In some systems it is taught that as individuated essence, we take on certain aspects of dis-ease and distortion, certain issues, to heal them in that lifetime – for one's own benefit, as well as for the benefit of all.

Back to the quantum universe: we are all connected in a quantum way and a certain action "here" will have effects "there". It really is spooky healing action at a distance.

For energy healing to "hold" for an individual, it can, nonetheless, be essential to bring awareness to the issues, to accept, assimilate and then allow the new, more integrated self to be. Otherwise, the energy flow will just keep running into the block again. We will, in most cases, either make a shift that is so profound that the old ways just won't be used, and/or have to build new circuitry. This takes awareness and practice.

Healing cannot happen without the agreement of the higher self of the individual.

Why I was called at this time is a matter of speculation, but not a surprise looking at what is happening all over the planet. I am simply agreeing to be available for holding the healing space and doing energy work for and with those who wish to receive it.

We are all somehow connected through a mechanism not currently, nor completely understood by science or the human mind. Changes, shifting and healing can happen, seemingly incomprehensibly, like in a miracle or by magic. One most important ingredient in healing is intention. But if you were raised Catholic, this saying should sound appropriate right here: Your belief has helped you. This belief is 100%, one of no doubt. Heart love, a love force from your heart, also heals.

Scientifically speaking, it still is a mystery and we can't yet explain how exactly distance healing works. This puts it still more in the realm of what could be called magic. Through the interplay of healer and participants, intentions, energy, plasmas and fields, plus the mysterious spooky action at a distance factor, healing at a distance plays its part in the healing for all of us.

There may be an even deeper way: accessing the state of being before manifestation, and manifesting differently.

Nobel Prize winning physicist David Bohm writes about the implicate order of the holographic universe, a concept suggesting that the entire universe is an ever-changing cosmic hologram that is layered with information. Because it is a hologram, every little part contains information about the entire universe. Each layer holds a higher order of information and each higher order is enfolded in an aspect of space/time. The higher order may be thought of as consciousness as it "descends" wave-like into form. Thus, consciousness is indeed in all things and causes all things.

Bell's Theorem provides mathematical proof of non-locality. I am not saying I understand the mathematics of it, but I am accepting what they say. If two photons are non-locally connected, communication between them can be instantaneous because they are not truly separate – information can be transferred faster than the speed of light. Though actually, I am not sure if transfer is even the correct term for it. Maybe those stories of Tom Brown Jr. being able to move objects in a room, even though he was physically far away, are actually true?

Bohm already suggested that at the subatomic level, all points in space are essentially the same, and therefore, nothing is actually separate from anything else. If we think about locality in terms of the particle (specific point in space) behavior of light, then non-locality can be seen in terms of light behaving as a wave where it is indistinguishable and interconnected.

Basically, what modern science tells us is that fundamentally, there are no separate parts to anything, and that everything is connected to everything else.

Sages of ancient times and prophesies have long told us this. Everything is energy dancing in form, going in and out from formless into form. Most humans have not yet grasped what that could mean for us as conscious beings. Observation also changes the observed, and even the terms past and future become something not fixed. Past events can be changed, past lives can be healed and it will have an effect for you now. There is also ancestral healing.

Bohm states that everything is non-locally interconnected and the world is an "unbroken wholeness". It really is all one. So in the most healed state, this is realized. I am not sure if you can see, sense or feel the mind-blowing potential this holds for the development of conscious beings and health and healing of these body-minds of ours. Atoms are made out of invisible energy, not tangible matter... and intention, consciousness, or whatever you call it, can change how it manifests. Can we allow ourselves to align with the highest vibrations to manifest the highest version of ourselves?

Maybe Tom Brown's story of "Grandfather" not actually dying, but dissolving into light at the end of his life is not just a story either?

Time is a function of space, and not linear. Spirit is senior to matter and modern science is catching up to that.

After all that, best I can tell, Distance Energy Healing works, or can work, because of the deepest nature of the universe.

"It is so important to not give yourself away to someone, to give away your own responsibility for driving your car, meaning your body, your mind, your emotions, your spirit."

~ E.J. Gold

What is High Sense Perception?

High sense perception is simply a way to say that something is perceived, not using what is usually considered the five senses: physical sight, sound, smell, taste and touch.

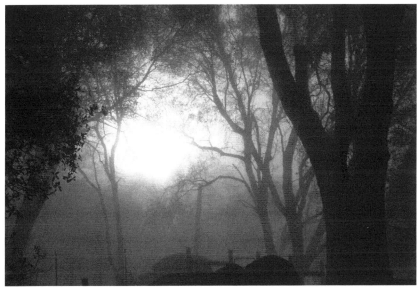

Gateway

Leaving proprioception alone for the moment, you might have heard of a sixth sense which usually refers to telepathy, seeing auras, clairvoyance, your mind's eye, picking up "vibes" off someone or a space, tingling, telepathic speech, direct knowing, kinesthetic perceptions. I know that Native Americans in California moved to high ground and warned the settlers about the storm that was to cause the great California flood. They just knew, and it was more than reading the clouds. They were tuned in and connected, whereas the settlers were not.

All these extra-sensory modes of perception are valid natural ways to perceive and communicate. Growing up in a very dense consensus reality that denies all of it, most humans, at least in our Western culture, never develop the skills. Not only that, often high-sense perception is denied or shamed or actively discouraged. There are, of course, especially gifted individuals, for whom Western culture cannot not suppress these skills, no matter what.

These days the army tries to train people to use their sixth sense, to be able to evade danger or act on something that cannot be proven or seen yet by technical instruments. Tom Brown Jr. has always said that in the end, mere physical survival skills will not be enough. The wandering groups will need spiritual means to be able to survive.

Even though high-sense perception skills are not commonly trained or taught, humans are naturally made for them. It just takes a willingness and practice as well as skill. Often there is fear or old mental or emotional baggage to clear, but anyone can learn high sense-perception and learn to trust it.

There are studies in some countries that examine DNA and the amazing possibilities still largely unexplored, such as there being tiny wormholes which connect to other dimensions.

But how do I know I don't just make it all up? Are my perceptions just imagination, made up stuff that I "see"? A very good question and one I have asked myself a lot, too. Often it is easier to discount perception or intuition. The more clear you are, the more pure in heart and intention, the more reliable your perception. This requires you to self-observe. If you are in a state of upset, anger or jealousy, your high-sense perception could be totally unreliable if you can even be there. It might not even come through with all the other internal "noise". And if it is there, you might put a spin on it that is just not objective. It just gets more and more subtle. Your random thoughts alone can interfere, and you will need to allow them without any kind of attachment or emotions put on them. In order to listen and see, there needs to be silence and a clear screen, as clear and quiet as you can be.

Having said that, perception of higher vibrational realities, nonetheless, will get filtered and processed according to who you are.

You will end up using words, when maybe a painting would be more appropriate. Painting skills could come in handy for those whose main perception skills are visual. In reporting, it is important to first learn to just perceive, as in just see or hear, without putting a spin or interpretation on it. As I write this, there is a tool developed by E.J. Gold that can help with that – the PLS course. What do you see? What do you know? What is the story?

At some point, your doubting mind will need some sort of proof that your perceptions in the higher realms are not all just made-up. How that happens is different for everyone. Here I will share another couple of examples of what I mean.

During one of the philosophy classes with Tom Brown Jr, we were doing some facing of the dark side. As usual, there was sharing after exercises or meditations. During one of those sharings, a bearded man, a lawyer from some state in the Eastern USA, talked about how he was facing a huge menacing form in the shape of an insect, that wanted to devour him. He was scared and didn't know what to do, until he decided to love it. He sent it love. (We had been taught that the dark side is only up to a certain level, and that beyond that, it cannot go. There was a meditation in that regards, too.) In any case, the huge shape, which looked about as huge as a blue whale, just in insect form, changed and was no longer menacing. It was transformed and he approached it. As I was listening to him tell the story, I could not believe my ears, because… I had witnessed the whole thing, just didn't share because, well, what if it was just imagined? I still had no faith that I actually had perceived it. Now, however, my experience, too, needed to be shared. Hopefully, for him, this was an equally confirming event regarding perceptions in the realm of non-ordinary realities as it was for me.

Another event happened during one of the BBSH homework healings I did, working with my housemate at the time, who was also a student. We had the table set up in the basement, which had a sliding glass door leading to a back patio. When I was doing the balancing and had arrived at the pelvic area, a dark hooded figure approached from outside and came through the door to eventually stand on the other side of the table across from me. At first I thought it was a monk, but it soon became menacing and with intent to kill. It got pretty scary when it raised an arm with a knife to plunge into the pelvis of the client. My two huge guides appeared, standing next and slightly behind me, one on each side, and telepathically talked me through it and told me what to do. One main thing was to stay grounded, focus, breathe, continue your work, keep the heart open and stay present with your client. Eventually, the figure dissolved and we finished the healing session. Later, on debriefing, she says she saw (in HER mind's eye) a dark shape entering through the door and approaching her.

With events like this, you eventually gain confidence. Also, as you pay more and more attention to that quiet inner voice of intuition and knowing – having disregarded it over and over, only to find out you were right on – you start listening to it and take appropriate action.

There are meetings in the spirit world, there are lucid dreams and there are states of actual transference of consciousness, a merging with another life form in a different time/space, including their perceptions.

How this confirmation of your high-sense perceptions happens for you, should you embark on this journey, will show up in your life the way you need it. You will also know how to deal with it. Trusting in your benevolent higher guidance and beings, or guardian angels, will be part of that process.

No idea, however good and accurate, will substitute for "personal experience personally experienced".

"Enlightenment is the first step on a very long journey."

~ E.J. Gold

The Healer Woman Soapstone Carving

In the announcement of the Distance Healing event, an image of a small carved soapstone figure, named Healer Woman, was included. Some called it politely: it won't read very well, and actually, maybe it is a pretty wretched carving. Yet, it signifies one of the most defining moments of my life. Here is the story, which I have never told to anyone before.

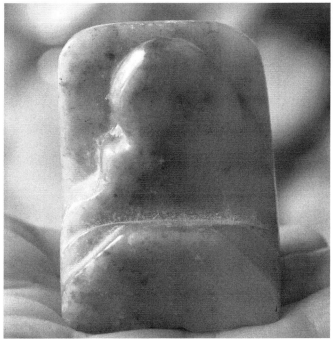

Healer Woman – Carved Soapstone

It was back in 1989, after I had started working as a Fellow at the Long Island Jewish Hospital in Queens, NY, that I took a trip on the LIRR (Long Island Rail Road) to Manhattan. There, in one of the bookstores, I saw this book: Tom Brown's "Field Guide to Nature and Survival for Children". I bought it.

There was nothing in that book I objected to and I became very interested. So I registered for the Standard Class, a survival class, a prerequisite at that time to taking any other classes in the Tracker School. It was a week-long adventure. The classes were still held at the farm in New Jersey in those days. We slept 50 people in the barn in a hay loft, some had brought tents, and in the daytime all of us downstairs crammed onto wooden benches during the lectures. We had survival tracker stew all week. I won't go through the stages I went through in relation to the teacher, but at the end of the week one thing was crystal clear to me: I would go to the philosophy classes, and I did, to several.

As an aside, there was a fairly large Native American type sweat lodge on the premises, and I participated in one led by Tom. Periodically, the door would be opened and I remember one of the things he said during that first and only sweat lodge I experienced at the Tracker School: "Let the healing begin." That is when my conscious healing began.

I learned many things during my times at the Tracker School that stayed with me through the years, in fact, even decades later, when some things became clear to me in a different way other than mental knowledge, I would remember: "Tom said that years ago… THAT is what he meant!" Even something I encounter working in the garden these days – I still remember a particular lesson regarding saplings and finally am understanding what he had meant. I understand it now because I am there, at that level, where it makes sense this could be an issue. Before then, I heard it, took it in, but didn't really know/feel/understand what the "issue" was, because I was not there, and did not have the experience.

I don't recall if it was during the first or second philosophy class where the soapstone carving came in. Before I go there, let me tell you something Tom told us at an earlier class, paraphrased here: "You come here from all walks of life, trained and steeped in the Western culture. You don't have to believe anything I say. I am not trying to change any of you or take any of what you have learned away. What I am asking is this: For this one week, allow yourself to play, just put all that you know on a shelf and allow yourself to play. And see what happens."

That made sense to me and I was willing to do it. As I am writing this, I am reminded how much got transmitted during the times and classes with him. In any case, here is what happened:

At the beginning of that week-long class, each of the students got a piece of soapstone rock and we were told to work on it during the week and carve something out of it. All week, including at the lecture times in the cramped rustic classroom, our hands were working on it, and mine did too, unless I was taking notes. There always was physical work with the hands during the classes. The "carving" tools I had were my little survival knife and sand paper. And how I tried to get something sculptural out of that soapstone. Some folks there were producing little masterpieces, my sculpture was nothing like it, but I tried.

Meanwhile, we were taught a system of meditation and how to access various realms, subconscious, unconscious, past and future times, then entering the spirit world and from there opening the doors to the higher levels of the spirit world, including the level where healing happens. Beyond that, there is the layer of the dark side and later, the levels where only love/light can exist, then the force that moves through all things, the creator and finally the void.

We went to journeys and did exercises and afterwards, students were invited to share their experience. Tom says this is because a success of one is the success of all of us. In time, we all would have something to share.

As the week went on, we went into meditations and took our soapstone with us. We didn't even take it into the spirit world, but to three distinct stations on the stairs down to that realm. At one station, we were to "see" the item, another to hear its sound, and an other to feel it. Truth be told, I don't really recall the third one for sure. To this day I remember what this carved soapstone sounded like, but most of all, what it looked like (in my minds eye during the meditation).

But then, one can imagine lots of stuff, right?

Okay, so now comes the end of the week, the very last day. We are sitting there in the morning with our soapstones. Then Tom held the item of each of the students in his hands for a moment.

Then we gathered just outside the barn. We could see two tables some distance away and apart from each other. We placed our carved stone on one of the tables and then went back to the barn entrance. There, we had to blindfold ourselves, to assure that our physical eyes were not used.

We got turned around a few times. Then this: The helpers would either leave the stone where it was, move it but leave it on the same table, or, move it to the other table.

We were to find our carved soapstone while blindfolded.

So I stood there, and "looked" in the direction of the table, "leftish" to me, not straight ahead, where I had placed it, but I could not "see it" or sense it there. I turned to the other table and got a yes in my gut. I did this three times before I concluded that: it had been moved to the other table. So I stood there some more, "looking" blindfolded at the other table. And I asked it to reveal itself. I stood there, and then, I SAW IT. It looked exactly like I had seen it (energy/light) during the meditation. Then, a light beam - the circumference of a common household broom handle - came, almost shot out, from the center of the item in a straight line to my heart, or maybe just a little underneath the physical heart. All I had to do now was follow that line, which I did. When I got to the table, the side the item was on, I discovered that there were so many people there, it was impossible for me to get to it.

I walked around the table, now on the other side of it, still blindfolded, still seeing the object where it seemed to be. Eventually I reached with my right arm back across the table, my hand touching a much larger object and landing on a small figurine. I took it, lifted it up with my right arm, took off the blindfold with my left arm and it was "it". I still remember the sensation and the unbelievable disbelief of my mind. It could not understand that this had worked, that the hand actually landed on the physical object my "other" eyes had seen – no way, no way. However, the mind had been there, observed the whole process and it happened. For me, there was no denying it as I held the physical object in my hand.

That was the moment I became free to explore non-physical

realities. Blindfolded, with my high-sense perception, I saw the energy form of a physical object and was able to find it, with a strong connection, and picked it up physically. From that day on, I was no longer bound by certain limits of Western society and traditional science. I knew there were more than the five senses we are taught about. There was another realm and a way to perceive it. And anyone can learn it.

The carving, wretched as it may look to some, is that of a seated woman. She has longish hair. She is a healer, through both energy and plant medicine, benevolent and welcoming, open armed, loving. The figurine is imbued and charged from that time and the years it was sitting on altars and in my healing room.

You might ask why I didn't stay with that school. The answer is: I realized I needed other work. Much later, in 2002, going back was one of the considerations for the next step on my path, but I was guided instead to work with IDHHB, the Institute founded by E.J. Gold.

Anyway, this is the story I never told before. The stone and my path are deeply connected, and it was one of the most important, and indeed pivotal, experiences of my life. No longer was it all just play and imagination. There is a world beyond our usually seen or heard consensus reality and we can perceive the non-physical energy forms. And I held the proof in my hands.

She has been part of my altars every since.

"Now is the time to get it right, clean up the mess, unscramble your life and put it in order. Only then can you fully address the deeper matters of spirit."

~ E.J. Gold

What Will You Be Doing?

During our first introductory Distance Healing event on gorebaggtv, someone asked what I would actually be doing.

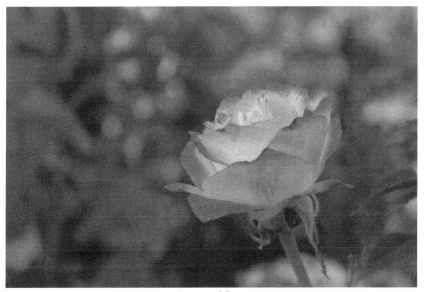

Inner Glow

"Things do not change; we change."

~ Henry David Thoreau

Here is, in brief, what I actually do.

I prepare for the event and set up the altar. We open the livestream, then do the mic check, greeting, answer questions, relaxation and invocation, open the healing space, hold the space, do energy work as it shows up, observe, listen, close the space, write the notes, post the notes. During the time that the music plays, for about 40-50 minutes, the energy work happens. I am available to do energy work for anyone who asks. To answer what I then actually do, it helps to know the following:

As all beings, humans have an energy field associated with their body. There are various layers to this field. Energy blocks in the energy field can lead to dis-ease, either physically, mentally, emotionally or spiritually. Energy blocks can occur on any level of the field. With high-sense perception, energy is perceived, energy blocks can be charged, loosened or removed. Most of the time, energy gets channeled from the ground up and through the hands. Sometimes a general charging and cleansing of the entire field is asked for. Sometimes chakra work needs to happen, or work on the level of intention. Sometimes re-connection and remembering on a soul level is needed. I use high-sense perception, my hands, hara or the level of intention. Sometimes guidance will come through which I will speak or let you know later in the write-up posted online. Those for whom it is meant will recognize it and know.

When there is no specific request, the energy just automatically goes where it is most needed. That extra charge can be all that is needed to get things moving.

When energy blocks are removed from the energy field, healing can happen suddenly, or gradually, as physical dis-ease no longer has a foothold and will cease to manifest.

Here is an example. During my time at BBSH, the class was going to do healing with guides. I don't know if we were late or what the reason was the other person and I not to get a chance to talk about anything prior to the start of the session. In any case, I was being the healer and when, during the chelation, I reached the pelvic area, I saw a dark shape in the uterus, about the size of a large walnut. I held my post as the two guides came in and did what they do – surgery to remove it. All I did was hold still and they used my arms as a vessel. After they were done, I continued the chelation. At the end, on debriefing, she could not believe it. At first when she noticed I stopped at the pelvis, she thought: "No, I already have an appointment to remove it", but then relaxed into it. After the healing, I found out she had been diagnosed with a tumor of some sort and surgery was to happen after class was over. She canceled the surgery, totally believing she would not need it, focused on being well and went back 3 months later and they could not find the tumor. Surgery was indeed not necessary.

The dissolving of physical manifestations might require your participation in some form, including awareness and recognition for a need to change the way you think or do some things in your life. It requires a listening deep within, to your higher self and being honest with yourself.

A certain amount of the time, during our online healing event, I simply hold the space, or access very high states of being, facilitating everyone to go there. Going into higher states of being is not to be underestimated in the process of healing and transformation. The more often you go there, the higher the chance for transformational change. In addition, accessing and being in higher states can lead to spontaneous changes that get expressed physically.

The Distance Energy Healing event is an opportunity to give yourself the gift of time, a time to connect with yourself and re-connect parts of yourself. It is a time for self-care and love, a time to breathe, raise your consciousness, trust and allow yourself to relax into a state where transformation and healing can happen on whatever level it is needed. Healing angels, higher spiritual beings and I are standing by to do specific energy work to aid you in that process, if you wish. I will be holding the highest vibrational space possible for the duration of our healing event. It is a time to connect with the highest and deepest part of who you are. A time to connect with the Divine.

"The ultimate metaphysical secret, if we dare state it so simply, is that there are no boundaries in the universe. Boundaries are illusions, products not of reality but of the way we map and edit reality. And while it is fine to map out the territory, it is fatal to confuse the two."

~ Ken Wilber

"Knowledge is a steady flow, not what you know."

~ E.J. Gold

The Lost Works

What Makes You Think You Can Do This?

If you have read the Distance Energy Healing or the Call, chapters, you will have an idea about how this offering of Distance Energy Healing came about, and why I think I can do this – to hold the space for the healing event and do some energy work during that time. For me, this is simply listening and following the call, accepting and surrendering to a higher will, trusting it is for the highest good.

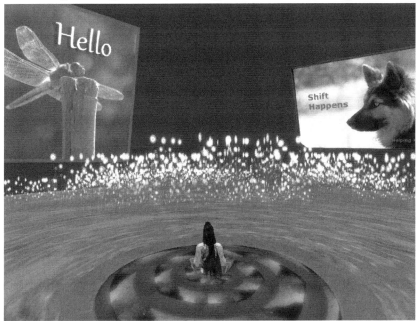

Hello – Shift Happens

However, there are other ways to look at the question, and this post is about that, not any type of credentials. There is the questioning and wondering, such as: If you "are a healer", then how come you react this way or that way, say this and that? Why don't you act more like one all the time, or at least, more often?

Actually, I am addressing this openly because of coming across a post on social media after someone I know published a very good and potentially hugely helpful book for many people on the spiritual path. What if, because of what was said, someone putting two and two together, would not read that book and start on a particular path? The book is excellent and inspired, as well as a reflection of deep dedication to this path. In any case, if I am holding the space as an energy worker, how come I don't do it all the time? How come I can act like such a bitch/asshole (according to some)?

"You are here to learn to pass on to a higher level, not here to learn how to die and get buried in the dirt."

~ E.J. Gold

"Be the most ethical, the most responsible, the most authentic you can be with every breath you take, because you are cutting a path into tomorrow that others will follow."

~ Ken Wilber

"Don't be an end user"

~ E.J. Gold

First of all, I too, am still not done with my own journey – which continues till the day I die. I am whole only to the degree that I am aware of it. But to put a limit on it, no – this is a journey and remains one. In fact, I am embarking on a whole new stretch, and this is only the first step in it. While there is great uncertainty, there is also excitement about the possibilities.

Most of all, I trust the divine guidance. I believe in the healing power of presence, the source of all Being, to reconfigure us as needed.

An important credential in my own mind is the journey I have been on in this life, the depths and darkness faced and traversed and submerged in, the work done and methods tested and explored, the passages gone through, to come out more and more whole, wiser and open-hearted.

This is gonna be a possibly sobering post that will, however, help with any projections that might be floating around in the field, as in: I have no aspiration to be anyone's great healer upon which you project any special qualities. Know that qualities you project onto others, both the dark and the golden ones, are really your own. The space of the Distance Energy Healing event is a shared sacred space we all create, with me only having a certain function in it. The healing energies don't originate in me, they flow through me.

I would like to recall something that happened at the Barbara Brennan School of Healing.

It was Sunday evening at the initial orientation/greeting space. The teachers would go, one by one, up on the podium to introduce themselves. There was one striking woman teacher in her fifties who got up there and said: "I don't want to be here." She then went on to say a few other things, none of which I remember, other than her honesty. I felt such a relief and thought: yes, I am in the right school if someone can say this.

She did not even work with first year students, but to this day, the event she held was the highlight of every week for me for the next two years. Then she left the school after about a decade having taught there. She and her husband were offering the "Temple of the Beloved" four times a year.

After graduating, I worked with her by phone and eventually went to see her. During one of the sessions, I told her I so appreciated her honesty at the introduction, and she said something like: "Oh really, I got so much flack for it… but one just never knows…"

For me, or maybe just generally people of my type, the honesty of it was one of the most important things and started me off trusting. It made her "real" from the start and the school trustworthy in my eyes.

So what makes me think I can do energy work and healings when I have been called: selfish, cruel, an asshole, crazy, sick, jealous, a bitch and you know, things like that. Nevermind that some of that was projection. I also am not afraid to swear. Why would anyone in their right mind think that is a trustworthy person or being?

Two reasons: After my own journey and training, I can leave it behind, drop it, be a professional. Secondly, you trust yourself.

I actually have thought, felt and spoken in reactive or unkind ways, had to face those things many times in myself, starting as a very young child. In addition, it became clear to me in the early '90s that I had what appears to be a lifetime where I used dark magic and I'm still paying for that one. I learned the necessity of 100% focus and intention with every fiber of your being for certain effects to occur, and I was tempted, but knowing the utter futility, I finally said and meant it: I'd rather die than use it. That was the end of it.

There were many issues and I had to get to the core of and face, often repeatedly, just on deeper and deeper levels, including why I hated so often and with such deep rage and why the base note of my life was such profound sadness. It was a very very long journey to get back to any semblance of connection to self, to a somewhat integrated, grounded self. This life's journey got off to an early start with a profound shock-trauma lasting several weeks during early infancy, and then went on in other ways all through childhood. But the perinatal and first three months set a Do, a base tone and configuration, a start that is almost impossible to address as it is so pre-verbal and global. Yes, it already was a reflection of a deep soul issue. And, the fundamental neuro-circuitry of the then-developing organism was influenced and wired in such a way that affects me to this day. It is almost like a handicap one learns to live with unless and until rewiring happens.

I still have little tolerance to be around many people for a very long time, or maybe I should qualify – BS superficial type interaction and

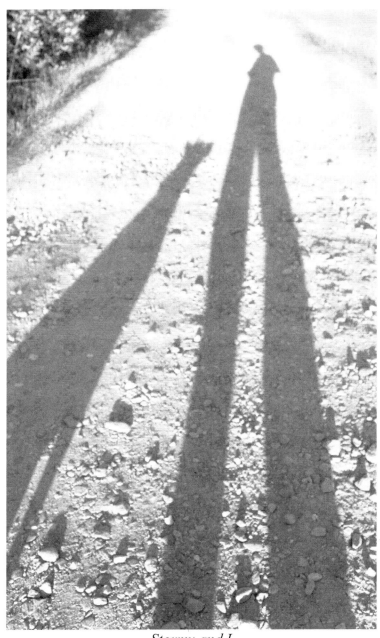

Stormy and I

social contexts. But no matter what, I need alone time, my own space… and it may have been crazy to put myself in a place where that is the one thing hardest to come by. But then, maybe that was part of my schooling and task in this lifetime.

While I have started a new phase in my own development, it has been difficult to get some rewiring done and some of the neuro-circuitry remains or defaults into a very early one. It usually takes intense presence to not react, and my deepest default to this day is to leave, if not physically, then internally. My brother, who I am "quantumly" connected to, said it like this: "I am struggling through life with my personal deficiencies", and I understood what he meant. I also know it is time for yet another change. This is a quantum universe after all and spirit really IS senior to matter. And then there are encounters with the divine – IT is calling me. So here we are.

In medical practice, I was well-trained and very good, with excellent clinical acumen. In healing practice, I am a pro with decades of deep personal and transformational work and training behind me. Energy work requires a certain state of being. I know how to hold healing space, know how to access a state of compassion and loving-kindness, I access core essence, limitless space and perceive in subtle realms.

Are there "better", more advanced individuals in the healing professions? You bet. Way better by my own estimation. I am offering the online healing hour and this book because I can, was called and because there are people who will be helped by it. It is possible I will at some point available be for working with individuals. At this time, there are other projects that are taking up the time.

Another important aspect for me is high ethics. Some of it got taught at home. I realized ethical dilemmas and a dark side inside myself in kindergarten at age 5 or 6, so that line of development seemed right on track. The BBSH as well as Hakomi teaches with high ethical standards, the spiritual teachers I worked with have high ethics. I simply would not even attempt to do certain types of work unless I can leave what is called in the pathwork "the lower self" behind for that time.

If you go to the doctor and he/she is so nice and professional, do you really think they always have that hat on at home or when out with friends? Maybe they just need to be who they are sometimes and maybe shit hits the fan at home occasionally, or a melt down happens?

It is kinda like that. Even on crappy days, do you act the same in the office as you do at home? Most people don't, and even though you might not see a huge difference, the way things are currently, there still is a higher state reached during the energy healing times than what is my everyday norm.

In any case, the other question that is looming in the air is this: how come you didn't do this all along? It is so needed in this world. You were doing it before, 14 years ago. Well, when I moved across the USA (which was a bardo trip into a new life) to California, I moved from a five bedroom house, with guest room, healing room, two rooms for a housemate and friend, to a shared household with not even a room to myself. It was very interesting to see many issues of my birth family repeated, in fact, that is how it became obvious that it was a lifetime within a lifetime. I started off being radiant (so I was told), but after two weeks, stuff started to happen. These days I am grateful to have the top of a bunk bed to rest on, and a desk with a computer. I have (volunteer) work in a spiritual community, and I don't even care if it is *in* the Work or *for* the Work. My real work is internal, expressing outwardly as this.

No one who has not lived like this can imagine the stresses and toll that it took, and for myself, at some point the physical pain got so bad and there was so little energy that I was starting to investigate medical cannabis. Alas, this god-given, sacred, medicinal plant is still not legal enough to just grow and juice, like you can with cabbage. However, the body needed attention and there was nutrition, juicing, stretching, nature and certain meditative practices and, backed against a wall, I changed some things I do, which was effective, and here we are.

Over the years there have been shocks, huge awakenings and permanent shifts. And presently I am intending to embody the best version of myself in whatever situation arises, even if it does not include any "luxuries". In fact, a few years ago while doing a cleaning job in the garden, I stacked some cement blocks and the result reminded me of "favelas" - a slum habitation - in Brazil. I modified it with some plant pots and concluded then: you don't need to be rich to do certain types of work. You can always do something. You don't have to litter. You can care for your surroundings and yourself. You can meditate and pray.

Being kinder and gentler in everyday interactions under extreme stress will probably remain a challenge, however, especially when I cannot take care properly (by my standards) of the animals I caused into being or have accepted 100% responsibility for. I know things are off if I am impatient with the nails and the hammer. These days I often remember enough to say "ayaya", rather than "fuck fuck fuck"… but to me, fuck is just a sound and does not have the qualities that native speakers attribute to it emotionally. (We did not swear, gossip or call people names at my house growing up – the worst it got was something in the form of a remark – *so ein scheiss aber auch*. I would hesitate to swear in German. Actually, I don't).

So many times in my life I wanted to just not be here any more, though when I was 16, getting up and having stepped onto the carpet, walking between the bed and my desk, some fraction of a second flash occurred and I knew I would not actively kill myself, that it was completely pointless. At the time I had no plans for it and wondered what it was all about. I also always stayed away from drugs as I knew I would not have it in me to ever get off them. In any case, since I started the spiritual journey deliberately, when the going got toughest, it is always this: I chant a Native American chant taught to us by Tom Brown Jr. – a chant to never finish to the end unless real help is needed – to call on the spirit guides to help me and guide me. And even during the worst times, it ends here: "Place me where I can serve the best, for the benefit of all beings". I cultivate that attitude, for it to hopefully remain in my conscious energy form after I die.

Not sure if this helped, but it was meant to let you know that someone can do a healing job, hold space and still be reactive or act like an ass (no offense to any animals) at other times. It gets better though, and we are just now entering a whole new evolutionary phase of what is possible in human incarnation, with more power, options and a much bigger, open heart.

These days I find myself walking up the driveway, thinking and feeling 'I am Home'. It is wonderful.

Everyone is on their journey to complete their mission for this life, this physical incarnation, this particular Earth game. Let's not forget to dance and play, and be kind to ourselves and others.

56

What Does Healing Mean?

Basically, healing is the process of becoming whole, or, more correctly – the process of realizing your wholeness.

Before going further with the question of what healing means, one might wonder: Why heal at all? Can't we accept how things are now, how the world is now and how we are now?

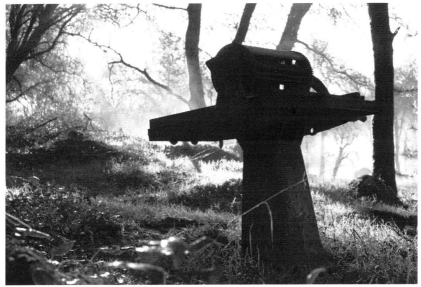

Blissful Morning upon the Rusty

Yes, there is an "enoughness" and perfection in NOW and what is happening, that would make healing unnecessary. Everything is indeed just as it is and it is perfect. That is one side of the coin and if you bring all your presence and attention to the NOW, you'd be well off. That is, however, not where you might find yourself, and there are many modalities or healing work that we humans may need on our way to becoming whole, or even functional, in life.

People are on various stages of growth and development. They are of different types and there are different kinds of trauma impacting us on various stages in life. Likewise, there are many levels and layers of healing.

In order to understand energy healing, it helps to be aware that humans are made of energy in the form of various bodies, from the physical, emotional, to various levels of energy bodies and the soul level.

Let's see: say you have a toothache – you ignore it as long as you can, but it is now starting to quite interfere with your ability to function. You are not a bad person, it is fine, and at some point you will take steps to get it handled. Some physical ailments really need the attention of the medical system.

Or, there has been a lot of stress in your life, and you feel out of whack, your back hurts more each day and you start to be very very grumpy. At some point, you decide to go see your acupuncturist to re-balance your energy, take some herbs and start doing exercises for your back.

You have a bad belly ache, nausea and vomiting – hm, this does not make you a bad person either, but you decide to get a medical opinion and next thing you know, you are diagnosed with appendicitis.

Energy work is like that, too. If there are blockages in the energy field, or there is a lot of "crud" in there – it can lead to psycho-emotional and physical symptoms, dis-ease, which makes it difficult to do what you need to do. So you decide to get some re-balancing and charging of your energy field. That will make it easier for your body to self-heal.

You have been told by the doctors that there is nothing they can do. You are working with alternative medicine – but now, you ask others to pray for you.

Maybe you have been diagnosed with PTSD or complex PTSD, and nothing helped but a therapy dog to get you back on track.

All these measures are to restore your health and well-being. While these days most people associate healing with the physical body, the most profound is often the restoration of a sense of wholeness in the spiritual sense.

Please take a moment to reflect: What does healing mean to you? What images come up for you when you imagine healing?

In your view – is there a difference in the common meaning of being healthy vs. being whole? You can speak it: "I feel healthy", pause, then "I feel whole" – does it feel the same or does it mean the same to you?

The word "heal" comes from the word "hal" – and whole, holy, heal, heil all have the same Indo-Germanic word origin.

Healing means to make whole, becoming whole. It is a process of restoration of physical and spiritual integrity from a state of suffering, fragmentation or illness. Being whole, being healed, implies a non-brokenness, a non-fragmentation, an integrity, which then allows for functioning at the highest level that it can be. Some consider this really the essence of it.

To heal is to make/become whole, to re-integrate disowned parts into who you recognize as "you" and to enable energy to flow freely.

For a certain level of functioning on any given level of being, certain degrees of **wholeness, integration and consciousness need to be there**, and if that is not yet the case, healing may need to happen. Healing may be needed in Growth and Transformation.

You could find yourself doing well for a particular stage, place and time, and then, in your growth process, find that more integration, or a higher degree of healing, wholeness and integrated beingness is necessary to function at the next level. This movement into a higher level often is accompanied by a more or less rocky period in which "you" die to the old level only to reassemble, reintegrate yourself on the next higher level, ultimately, to include more and more of yourself until there is nothing excluded.

We – humans, our bodies – are built for healing and we are capable of transformation. Healing is taking on a whole new meaning in this age of science and spirituality coming together. No longer is "fixing" the body the only goal. In fact, many modern ailments are not "fixable" by traditional pill-oriented medicine.

In this age of humanity, it is time to "level up", to speak with gaming language, to make it on the planet. And those of you who are gamers, you know going to the next level means: coming to terms with the final level "boss monster". That is a struggle our world finds itself in these days.

Of course, one could go to consciousness first and, since spirit is senior to matter, go from there. In any case, to be better equipped for the happenings of our times, we may need to level-up.

Healing is necessary on a global level and in many aspects of our now antiquated and partly obsolete cultural establishments, and healing starts within each one of us.

How can you heal the outer when the inner is fragmented, unconscious and disjointed? Healing methods are numerous, and which one you may need, no one knows better than your inner self. Working with healers, spiritual guides, alternative medicine practitioners and methods, dreams or journaling along with traditional Western medicine, is becoming more accepted these days.

Even as a new level of healing is emerging with the evolving of conscious embodiment and awakening, holistic healing is a very old concept which got a bit lost in the rise of Western civilization and mindset.

Healing may need to be physical, emotional, or on various levels of psychological and energy fields. It may be needed in the thinking process and belief system. And it includes the spiritual aspects of a being. Dreams often reveal parts of ourselves that lie in the unconscious, waiting to be integrated into the whole of who we are. Even everyday dreaming is essential to our health and well-being on many levels.

Some of the descriptions that follow might make you think of a modern day spa, and in fact, even more inclusive.

In ancient Greece, people would go on a pilgrimage to the healing sanctuaries of Asclepius, the Greek God of Healing. Those sanctuaries could be found all over the Hellenic world. This tradition was active for almost 2000 years starting from around 1300 BC. In those healing sanctuaries, there would be the offering of bodywork, hydrotherapy, psychotherapy, good food and changes in diet. People going there also enjoyed theater, music and poetry, which can touch on a very deep soul level and thus, provide healing. When the temple "Therapeutes" (therapists) considered a person was ready, they would be introduced to the Abaton. The Abaton was a space where the patient would pray and sleep – expecting a visitation from Asclepius in their dreams. Healing would come about through the appearing of the healing god (or one of his totems) in a dream. Often the dream would result in a spontaneous healing or provide an indication of what needed to be done or undone for healing to occur. Please make a note of what "body" the patient was most likely using to meet the healing god.

Isn't that all amazing? This particular description sounds quite contemporary to the 21st century. Much has been written in books and on the web on healing modalities of all sorts. In recent years, many high tech devices have been added, as well as color, light and vibrational modalities for healing. In addition, research in neuroscience is coming up with astounding results. There has been research into meditation and brain changes, nutrition and the microbiome and so much more. We'll be exploring some of those in the course of an adventure elsewhere. I just thought I'd introduce the general concept of "healing" here.

You may have heard of the placebo effect, where people get better because they think they are getting medication. That is the same as saying: your belief has helped you.

Here is THE most important part of healing: awakening. It all is, in the end, a matter of consciousness and energy. There are simply many ways to do it and sometimes the path is littered with many little awakenings, sometimes there are very major events, and sometimes it is both. One ingredient is necessary: you have to want it. Your being has to agree. And let those sleep who don't want to become aware.

Some souls come in with a certain wholeness, others need to first do what might be called "soul" retrievals.

How can you be whole without including all parts of yourself? And how can you include all parts of yourself without being aware of them? Yes, exactly. After a while, the self you are aware of just gets bigger and bigger, more and more inclusive.

Growing up Catholic, I remember this: what you have done to the least of my brethren, you have done to me. Today what this means to me is: it is ALL God, the body of Christ – and anything done to anyone, to all sentient beings and to anything anywhere – is done to G*D.

Love your neighbor as your Self – not like you would love yourself... but AS your Self... because they are your Self... as is everything and everyone... the universe still is all One. And it is all prefect.

When working with a healer, or sacred circles and ceremonies, there is often the possibility to experience high states of being through deep relaxation and resonance.

Even if you think all of the universe is a mathematical something or other, a game or a sim, healing methods still apply. Within the game, you can rewrite your own programming.

If you are a Labyrinth Reader and also look at what modern physics is telling us: it really all is swirling patterns of light in infinite extension, forever waves unless observed and the observer determines the state of the particle. Have we begun to see what that could mean?

I am lucky to be able to use the transmitting services of the Institute for the Development of the Harmonious Human Being, IDHHB. Initially, I took that name to mean: to develop into a harmonious human being – which is perfect for healing. It also means the further development once you already are a harmonious human being. Growth and learning does not stop.

It takes, or rather, for a lot of folks it takes a lot of work to recognize the embeddedness of our body-mind into the culture, family and schooling system. You can't really see it unless you finally get some distance, perspective, insight and then you can look back at it.

To treat the root cause of illness and energetic imbalances, energy needs to move. It is crucial to move stuck energy, and energy work/healing is just one way to do this.

Given what is coming to light these days regarding the DNA, quantum physics, parallel worlds and multiverses and the whole idea of integral practice, the development of humans that is possible might be pretty much unexplored and unimaginable at this time. Part of the healing process is simply becoming a harmonious human being. From there, possibilities appear to be mind-blowing. You will need to learn to

62

vibrate with different frequencies, higher frequencies. You will need to monitor and yes, change the thoughts that lower your frequencies.

Here is a little exercise you can do. Rate how well you feel on a scale from 1-10. If the number is less than 8, recall the thought you were having just before that. Now think of something you love, uplifting, like that. Now rate your state again. Any difference? Next step: really feel that higher vibrational thought manifest in your body. Let your body partake in it. Now rate how you feel. Keep practicing, experimenting on how thoughts affect your well-being. It is, and always has been, about vigilance, observation, willingness, relaxation and practice, practice, practice.

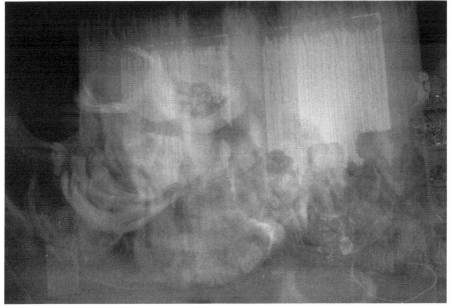

Movement

Energy Healing can get things moving, removing the foothold for physical ailments, and it still takes your self-knowledge and attitude and willingness to change more permanently towards a healthier, more whole and vibrant you. You want it to stick. In the end, you will need to learn to manage the energy you are, and this includes your body, thoughts and feelings. To build new internal circuitry might be needed to manifest a more whole you. It will not only require your participation, it will require you to become totally responsible.

Just as it took many repetitions to build your first habits, it will take many repetitions to replace them with other, healthier default pathways.

Western medicine does not help you discover where your greatness lies or invite you to go to the next level of what you are capable of.

In your healing, you will need to become responsible and take care of all aspects of your self, asking for and getting help when needed.

I am providing a weekly online space where you can start or deepen your journey.

For some, healed means to be truly home, to be one with the source of all, to have realized your true nature.

"Health is a state of complete physical, mental and social well-being, and not merely the absence of disease or infirmity."

World Health Organization, 1948.

From the internet:

heil

das Wort geht zusammen mit

got.*hails,* altengl. *hal* und altfrz. *hal* auf germ.**haila–* „gesund, ganz" zurück; außergemanische Verwandtschaften lassen auf eine gemeinsame indogermanische Wurzel **koilu–* „gesund" schließen; das Substantiv
Heil weist trotz der gleichen Lautung keinerlei Verwandtschaft zu *heil* auf; es geht auf ahd. *heil* zurück und ist verwandt mit
altengl. *hæl* und altfrz. *hel* „Vorzeichen"; in den altnordischen Sprachen existierte zunächst noch ein weiteres Wort gleicher Lautung mit der Bedeutung „Glück, Segen"; die beiden Wörter sind dann ineinander übergegangen.

Healing, noun, adjective. … **Word Origin** and **History** for heal. v. Old English hælan "cure; save; make whole, sound and well," from Proto-Germanic *hailjan (cf. Old Saxon helian, Old Norse heila, Old Frisian hela, Dutch helen, German **heilen**, Gothic ga-hailjan "to heal, cure"), literally "to make whole" (see health).

In Hebrew, the word for dream is halom. According to some scholars, the verb (halam), "to dream," and the verb (halam), "to be in good health," are related.

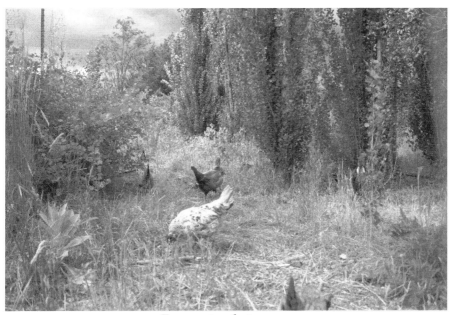

Expressing beingness

"The wound is the place where the Light enters you."
~ *Rumi*

"Real change comes from repetition."
~ *E.J. Gold*

"To understand the whole, it is necessary to understand the parts. To understand the parts, it is necessary to understand the whole. Such is the circle of understanding. We move from part to whole and back again, and in that dance of comprehension, in that amazing circle of understanding, we come alive to meaning, to value, and to vision: the very circle of understanding guides our way, weaving together the pieces, healing the fractures, mending the torn and tortured fragments, lighting the way ahead—this extraordinary movement from part to whole and back again, with healing the hallmark of each and every step, and grace the tender reward."

~ Ken Wilber
The Eye of Spirit

Methods Of Healing

Healing, becoming whole, easing suffering – how is it done?

There are many methods that can be useful in that regard. Methods will vary depending on where you are at in life and your development and who you are. Some methods are dictated by cultural beliefs and practices. What follows in the listings below are mostly methods employed in personal healing journeys for people in the Western culture which, with travel opportunities and information available from all over the world, include systems of healing from other regions the world.

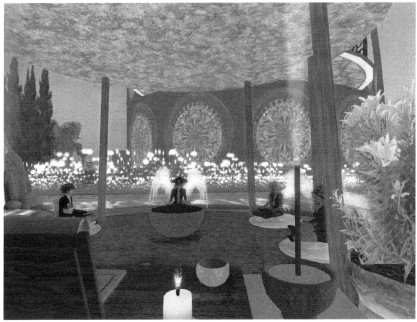

Online Meditation - Prosperity Virtual Ashram or PVA

Fundamentally, our bodies are energy and awareness/consciousness. That is not a very practical way for most people to look at it, but it is something to keep in mind.

The Western medical system does not teach you about radical self-care, it does not teach you how energy moves through your body and how it gets stuck, leading to illness. Western medicine does not teach you about food as medicine or herbal remedies. Western medicine does not teach you the importance of grounding, poetry and art, it does not teach you about finding your soul's purpose, or seeing illness and obstacles as gateways to a higher form of you.

However, in case of a serious accident, I'd recommend rushing to an emergency room, they know what to do. Got a life threatening bacterial infection? Even with emerging resistances due to antibiotic overuse, there still is a good chance they can save you. Need to temporarily be on life support – they can do that, as well as replace joints, provide prostheses, open clogged heart vessels, repair brain aneurisms, do gene therapy, organ transplants and more. In case you need measures that drastic, yes, you can be in good hands.

When it comes to attending the spiritual dimension, your connection with the Divine, seeing you as a whole, Western Medicine is not doing so hot. And maybe it is not meant to, but we really need to accept its limited role and function and take charge of the rest of who we are.

I will give you a few general pointers: bodies tend to self-heal – this is potentiated by loving and supported by giving it the right foods and plants. Epigenetics, a fairly new emerging field in biology and medicine, teaches us that certain experiences in life can turn genes on and off and lead to different expressions of our health, improve health or worsen it, depending. It is not new age mumbo-jumbo. Newer science tells us that what we believe, how we feel and interact with ourselves and our environment contributes to our health and well-being. What you believe does matter. We can access and change our unconscious beliefs and conditioning and change what we do and how we are.

Most of our programming has been put in before first grade. In the last decade or so it has become obvious that genes do not control our biology, but that perception of the environment does. Your beliefs are crucial in how you express health or out of balance being. DNA is your blueprint, but it is your nervous system that does the selection and expression of it/you. Your perception of the environment is crucial. The placebo effect really does work.

How transformation really gets stimulated and why people transform really is not known. Often the impetus is pain, but other times simply amazing experiences happen to put us on the road to transformation. Something much greater than us moves through it – and us all. Becoming aware, waking up, changing meta-habits and allowing different experiences can be healing. Self-knowledge is important, being connected and in your body is important. It will be difficult to change your body when you are not in it, when you are not grounded, when you don't care for it.

Intention and belief are very powerful. Stress management is helpful, supportive loving relationships are helpful, connection to the Earth is helpful and one of the best: mindfulness. All are helpful in the healing process. Practicing different thoughts is helpful.

The basics for health and healing can be kept very simple for all: belief that you are always healing, diet (real food), right exercise, connection to nature/body, mindfulness/meditation, being creative, playing with your thoughts and choosing the ones that raise your frequency, cultivating loving-kindness and compassion to self and others.

What you might aim for is to be a harmonious being, functional in your life and being able to fulfill your life's mission. A balance will need to be struck to nourish your body, mind, relationships and spirit. You will need to find a balance that is right for you between self-care, social life, work life and spiritual life. For some, this ultimately gets lived every day in an integrated way.

Fundamentally, the healing journey is an ever-increasing circle of awareness, inclusion and acceptance of Self, all parts of it, light as well as dark, physical as well as energetic bodies, mind and spirit. You will face this higher self and lower self, conscious, subconscious and unconscious aspects of your self. Self-observation is critical. You cannot heal if you keep pushing some parts of yourself away. Face it, embrace it, integrate it, transcend and move to the next level.

Some healing methods deal with the physical, some are psychotherapeutic and body-mind methods, some work with energy, some address the spirit. Some bypass those and deal with the recognition of your true nature… and then handle what needs to be handled. Some don't concern themselves with healing per se, but leave it up to you to do the work needed to be functional, no matter where you are at.

In the Western world, a certain method and approach to dealing with health issues was developed: allopathic medicine. In the Eastern traditions, a different approach is used. Both have priceless and valuable contributions to make. There are shamanic practices all over the world, and herbal medications. Prior to the current extinctions, there was a plant or plant combination for every ailment of the body. Unfortunately, one of the most healing herbs on the planet has been illegal for decades in this country.

There are methods of adjustments to the body, like acupuncture, chiropractic, physical therapy and massages, cranio-sacral therapies, Feldenkrais, Alexander Technique, Gokhale method and myofascial release, to name some. Then there are other body-mind workers that defy any category. During my time at BBSH (Barbara Brennan School of Healing), a guest speaker was giving a presentation to the class. Listening to the talk and watching the way he moved, for the first time in my life, I thought: this person is not from this planet. (I still think so.) In any case, I made up my mind right then to work with him. Luckily, two appointments were available on the same day a few weeks away, and I took the train up to New York City. One session was in the morning, the other in the afternoon. The sessions went deep, including the bone level. Prior to this day, when putting my feet together, my knees could never touch. The left leg was somehow misaligned from the hip. I wanted that realigned. He did, and it is holding to this day. I was there with it, but I still don't know what he did. I wanted to be able to do what he did and study with him. That never happened, and my life didn't even lead me there to deal with my back issues. Sometimes I wonder what would have happened, but in the forks of the roads in life, not all will be traveled. What this taught me, however, was this: even a long-standing issue with bones can be healed in one afternoon. There is an ingredient that came from me: trust and belief that it could be done, and then this skill of this being not from this planet – okay, he used methods of healing unknown to me.

There are energy medicine methods like Reiki, Brennan Healing Science, Core Energetics, Healing Touch, Prayer and some shamanic healers and mediums. There are psychics. There are people that don't fit into any category. Did I mention Tai-Chi,Qi-gong, and Yoga?

I worked with someone over the phone for about a year while in the BBSH. She lived somewhere up North from me. I never saw her. One day, it was just before allergy season. I have had allergy symptoms ever since I moved to the United States. She said, you know you can do something about that. So in guided meditation I went into my DNA and changed it. That year, I did not have allergy symptoms. Were the trees not blooming that year? I don't think so. Was I imagining it? No, I was astounded.

Why am I mentioning these two examples? For one reason only: it is a testimony, which is third best. Second best is witnessing it for yourself. But nothing beats personal experience personally experienced. As with the Healer Woman soapstone figurine, these examples have one thing in common: I was totally willing to play with it, willing to put prior held beliefs on hold, willing to go with it, to trust. For me, those are not optional ingredients in healing, but necessary.

Also, in my life, I have been attracted pretty much only to people with high ethics and integrity. That helps. It is up to you to do your due diligence in that regard.

But, moving on with the list:

There are psychotherapies, mindfulness and meditation, flotation tanks and systems like the "Pathwork", healing relationships, gazing, healing art, dance and yoga, EFT (emotional freedom technique), Aka Dua, Hakomi, Matrix-Works, group work, recovery programs, trauma therapies, therapy animals. There are methods involving psychedelic substances. (Never tried those, any drugs, but some appear to be very awakening and have a healing effect).

Shadow-Work, or, making the hidden, dark or unconscious parts of yourselves visible and accepting and integrating them, is an important part of becoming whole. There is relational healing and sexual healing. Generational healing may need to happen - one amazing way is the Family Constellation Work.

Why generational healing? Because it affects you how your mother and grandmother and ancestors lived, what they thought, what habits they had. In my own life, it was not just having to deal with the gloom and guilt and shame of a nation called Nazis, but my mother, at age 7, lost her beloved father to the war. My grandmother lost her husband, her father, her mother, her brothers and uncles to the war, all in the same year. The family became the poorest in the village. My mother was closest to her mom and absorbed a lot of the emotions. And yes, it affected me deeply. Most of my life I would have described this as my baseline feeling/emotion: sadness, profound sadness, and most of my life I didn't know where it was coming from, until family constellation work and more recently validated in studies showing how mothers and grandmothers and lineage affect offspring.

Journaling and dreamwork can be an important part in your journey to wholeness. You might need to work with trauma or complex trauma and learn to engage your social nervous system. Sometimes working with plants and animals makes it possible to even begin to trust people.

Healing may need to happen in the collective of a people or group. Both atrocities suffered as well as perpetrated need to be faced, even if they lie decades or even hundreds of years in the past. These days social media can be important in that regard by bringing to your computer screen things you'd have lived in denial of all your life. Living in denial of a dark side only makes it come out in destructive ways.

There is nutritional medicine, mud therapies, Kneipp-Kur, sauna, ice and cold, earthing/grounding, light therapy, sound and vibrational therapy, aromatherapy. Healthy food is invaluable in supporting the body in the healing process. Not sure where sweat lodges fit in.

There are many many more methods that can be employed in healing, the process of becoming an integrated whole.

Is there a common thread? Yes, at some point it becomes clear to someone that there is an issue, a problem that you want to address and handle. Then you might be looking for and asking for help. Self-observation of the body, emotions and thoughts and repeated behavioral patterns are very important. Self-acceptance plays a huge role, as does beginning to self-care about body and mind, taking back your power and responsibility. There is care of relationships, to other humans and all living things, and the relationship to the Divine, the higher.

A lot of the above-mentioned methods involve other people, but there are many books and these days also a lot of webinars on the subjects. Some things get revealed and healed during your sacred times, meditations or a space where you feel safe.

It is no longer taboo to talk about the spiritual side of healing, awakening, the recognition that you are not just your body, but essentially a being of energy/light. There are healing paths with practices that incorporate mindfulness, self-observation, meditation, daily practices as main tools of awakening.

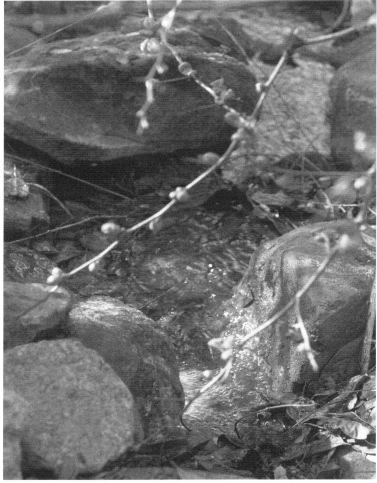

Spring

In case you expected a discussion of the pros and cons of a bunch of specific methods and therapies and who they are good for and such, sorry to disappoint you, but that is not a book I will ever write. I admire people who can do that. What I needed to get across is that there are many things out there to assist in your healing journey. It is up to YOU to investigate which ones are best for you, which ones you are ready for and engage in them, to pay attention which ones "coincidentally" seem to show up on your path. Get moving, free the energy and be in the flow.

Once you start the journey, the methods for you and your next steps will appear, and you then either engage them or not, as you are able, guided or drawn to. It is up to you to listen to your inner voice, do the due diligence and then choose the method you are drawn to. Trust your intuition, do what feels right. Some methods may serve extremely well at some point in your journey and development, then you outgrow them and need something else. That's okay and to be expected. Some practices stay useful through the course. In fact, pick a practice of some kind, even if it is only 5 minutes a day, but do it. If you want to be fast, let go of the beliefs that sabotage your manifesting your higher self. Remember, doing something fun, music and animals can help you to get rid of and manage your pain. Every morning, surround yourself with White Light.

Be kind to yourself in the process of your growth and transformation towards a more whole and integrated you. Really, be kind to yourself.

"There is no growth where there is no resistance."

~ E.J. Gold

Why I Left The Medical System

There is a very short answer to the question of why I left medicine, which hardly anyone understands, after all that training and such opportunities. I am not cut out to live and work as a physician in the system as it is currently practiced in the United States of America. As a kid, I wanted to go to Africa and help the children there. And a big part of me still just wants to do that, to help, specifically help people heal and become more aware from whatever point they are at. It is the pressures and demands of an abusive medical system that I am not cut out for. I have been called resilient by some, and fragile by others, and both are true. It did not help not having the proper life/work balance for a large portion of the time while working in medicine.

Don't get me wrong, there are a lot of very good, decent and well-meaning physicians and nurses, in fact, I never met otherwise, personally. But then, most folks in pediatrics might be different.

There are a lot of excellent parts to the current Western medical system in this country (USA), especially emergency and trauma care, some surgical specialties and procedures, organ transplants, hearing aids and, at least for those who can afford them, most of the very advanced cutting edge treatments, immune therapy or using DNA gene identification to customize nutrition or general care.

Still, most physicians were and possibly still are completely caught in a system they have grown up in, were taught in, and trust, a system that does not include other healing modalities. In addition, most have tens or hundreds of thousands of dollars worth of student loans and mortgages to pay and children to raise, plus, in some cases, the overhead expenses of a medical practice.

Even if one started waking up to what is not so good, and shocking even, there is no easy way out, even if you burn out or no longer agree with some of the premises, or the "standard of care". The suicide rate is not low, though not as high as that of veterinarians.

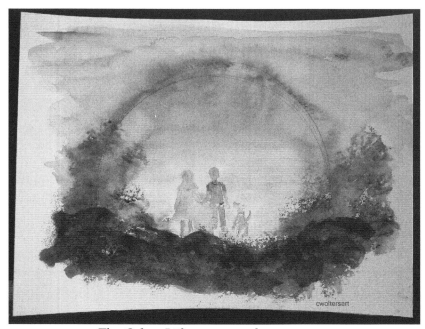

The Other Life – watercolor on paper

I went to medical school in Germany, where I grew up. University education is free there. Of course, taxes are a lot higher there, but the young are not the ones getting burdened. There, alternative ways of healing are widely accepted. Over 50 years ago my mom took my brother to a homeopath as the pediatrician said he didn't know what more to do. The homeopath did, and all was well soon thereafter. So I had that advantage: no cultural prejudice against non-traditional ways of healing.

After finishing medical school, I worked for the U.S. Army for two years. The first was at the Mannheim dispensary, then I transferred to the Station Hospital in Heidelberg, both urgent care and emergency medicine. Concurrently I studied for and passed the international exams to then do a pediatric internship (during which time I got divorced), and residency and neonatal intensive care fellowship in the USA. Because of visa requirements, I had to go back to Germany for two years, (good for family) and worked in a large children's hospital, getting to see the differences in medical practice close up. Some things were worse, some things better, some just different. One of the main differences: everyone had insurance. Back in those days at least, there were never ever considerations about whether or not some insurance would cover some treatment or another, or not.

As a doctor, I was very good at what I did, but once in general practice, I also realized how utterly devoid medical practice here was of any non-traditional ways of healing, how focused treatment was on "fix it", especially with antibiotics, which, when given without actually being medically necessary, cause not just unnecessary side effects, but can harm you by killing off all or most of the beneficial intestinal bacteria. Overall, the rewards of medical practice didn't make up for the negatives. I eventually started balking at more and more new vaccines being added to the infant schedule, some of which I did not consider necessary across the board for all infants and children. I had seen some of the devastating diseases that some vaccines protect from, and yes, I would recommend some vaccines, but enough was enough. Daily medical practice felt like an assembly line job. I loved the kids, but even they could not make up for the strain.

I realized that "nutrition" in this country puts toxins into children, obesity and related diseases were starting to skyrocket. And frankly, both parents working full time to just make ends meet, the low rate of breastfeeding (leading to the babies not getting the antibodies they needed) and having to put kids in daycare at two months of age, for crying out loud, where the babies of course ended up getting sick a lot – there was just no way. And, parents, you cannot hold your babies too much. All that leaving them and letting them cry it out and "teaching" them, all you are teaching them on a deep level is that their needs won't be met. Infants need your presence, and you need a support system for yourself if it is too much. But I digress. Large sections of the medical-pharmaceutical system here currently are misguided, though at the time I still had not realized it to the degree I do today. Still, there is something deeply wrong when so many kids get put on drugs for being "hyperactive", geez. One size of education does not fit all. And a lot of people just don't see it. And maybe the system just got worse, and with the current administration, things do not look better for the general population. But I digress again.

The lifestyle forced on doctors in the general practice specialties, and remember, this was over 20-30 years ago, felt abusive too. Pediatricians along with family physicians are at the low end of the pay scale to boot. In Germany, everyone gets six weeks vacation a year. Call is shared by citywide systems, where one is physically required about once every 6-8 weeks to participate, and gets paid for it. This does have disadvantages too, in terms of continuity of care. Every Wednesday afternoon all practices were closed for CME. Pharmacies were on a call schedule, too. Here, vacation time is two weeks, maybe three, plus a week for CME. And people here do not know any better. This life with two weeks vacation and a few holidays is just the status quo compared to Europe. In that regard, for physicians, especially in pediatrics, where over 50% are women now, things are getting better. These days they call it balance of family life and work life, and pretty much no physician still works the way I started out – on call every other night, all night and every other weekend, without the existence of cell phones and always within 15 minutes of the hospital because of availability for emergency c-sections. And honestly, some people can live like that and do well. I know one of them. The way I am configured internally was not compatible to keep it going. Even changing to every three nights on call and using a call service didn't help much, but it was a lot better.

By the time I went into private practice, I had been to Tom Brown's classes, started my own healing journey and was more consciously on a spiritual path. I went to study at the BBSH (Barbara Brennan School of Healing), also doing a few other things and the more I went into my own self-healing, the less I was able to stay in the system. I was not the same person that went into the field out of high school.

Add to that managed care, the constant looming threat of malpractice, the frequency of being on call, I finally changed jobs and went part time to pediatric Urgent Care for a large HMO for a couple of years. I still admire how some people are able to not only tolerate, but function well in the system. As a physician, I was good (excellent per someone else) but, when medicine became computerized with records requiring even more time at work with electronic "paperwork," I refused to see the same amount of patients as record-keeping took even more time. Well, that didn't go over well. By then, I had started locum tenens work, finished Hakomi training, my house was on the market. Ready for the next phase in my journey, I was on my way to California, planning on minimizing expenses, doing locum tenens for 3 months out of the year. But I ended up leaving medical practice. What remains is experience and informal consultations, or teaching. Especially in the years prior to the Affordable Care Act under Obama, some people without insurance would ask for advice and I'd tell them to go to urgent care or the ER if that seemed like the best route.

The thought of starting my own practice, fee for service and incorporating alternative medical healing modalities crossed my mind, but seemed unmanageable by the time I was ready to change my life, Actually, it was downright unrealistic.

There is yearly CME and I maintain one of 3 state licenses in case things in this country change in ways that require a return to some form of medical practice for some reason.

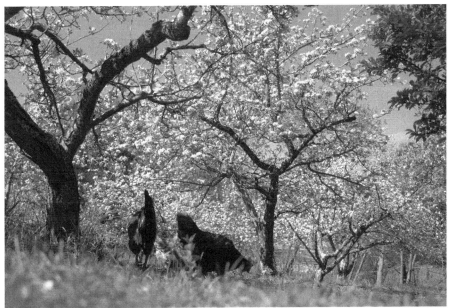

Natural Delight - Start living from a connected space

For the most part, Western medicine, as it is practiced today, treats symptoms. Medical doctors are not yet, and may never be, trained to address health issues holistically or working with the power of belief or patient's perception. Luckily, our bodies tend to heal if we don't interfere and keep making them having to deal with all the toxic stuff we ingest, inhale, see and expose ourselves to energetically. There is an innate intelligence in us that is a great healing force. Trust it and listen to your intuition about what is right for you.

I am where I am because of who I am and what I feel am able to do at this time. Some physicians in the system are worth their weight in gold. I admire them. I was not cut out for being such a doctor. But at my volunteer jobs, in very unrelated activities, some folks still call me Dok anyway.

I was called to offer help in the form of online Distance Energy Healing where all bring their own intention for healing, and to inspire you to take responsibility for your own health, well-being, life and transformation and learning to trust in the innate intelligence and force that moves though us all.

"Be the most ethical, the most responsible, the most authentic you can be with every breath you take, because you are cutting a path into tomorrow that others will follow."

~ Ken Wilber

Do You Trust "IT"?

When down by the chicken coops this evening, June 24, 2017, I kept wondering and thinking about a Facebook interaction.

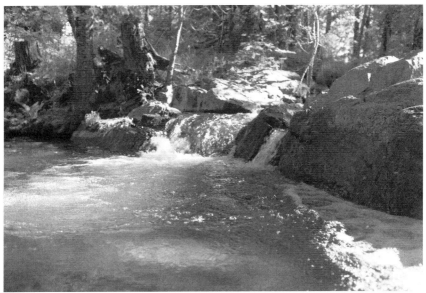

Bear River, California - Image courtesy of Karen Reif

Do you trust God's guidance? by Isabelle T.
In order to surrender to God, it helps to trust that this will create the highest outcome in our life.
Do you trust Spirit's guidance for you?
If yes, please share why.
If no, please share why.

I used to say: do you trust in Being… but my reply was:

Me: I don't call it God, but I trust it.

Isa: What do you call it?

Me: I don't actually… like I recently got "the call" (or another one)… and it just comes, I listen and do what is needed/asked for something like that…

Isa: I like that answer. As I create content for my course on "how to listen to '?'", I am filled with curiosity on how to use words to convey the unspeakable.

Me: I was just wondering about the naming thing… and… I am unable to name it… whatever name I came up with, was limiting "it". Divine guidance? Or maybe just guidance… but… not from a person or program… so how to convey the other kind…?

Isa: You just journeyed into my mind and heart! How to convey the unconveyable.

Me: Exactly.

When we say, "Do you trust the Great Spirit, the Spirit That Moves Through All Things, God, Allah, Being, the Absolute…?" It often comes with some cultural interpretation and limitation – too much for some. Any language will be limiting, and I like spirit/universe, but what I came up with was this:

I trust in what IS… the big ISNESS of all that is.

It moves, it knows and when there is, in humans, momentary or longer… non-resistance to movement (and it is not meant as physical movement) – non-resistance to ITs presence, when there is openness, willingness, then IT moves you. You really just are a being moved, as in taking appropriate right action, only at that moment there is no you. It is amazing how effortless it is, how there are no egoic considerations, how peaceful, how things just fall into place, there is energy and joy… but none of those terms feel as they used to.

Even if that which "I" ended up doing may later be judged by myself as "…oh, that is so little, not much, too ineffective", blah blah blah, at the moment IT moves through you… there is not so much guidance of a you, but rather IT is BEING YOU and IT knows all and flows in the way it needs to be flowed – through you – and we like to think of it as for the benefit of it/all.

It is beautiful.

It moves through all things and most creatures. It is the "conscious" creatures where potentially that flow gets thwarted and stuck. This is where the free will also comes in (though some schools say there really is no such thing as free will). The beauty of it is that those creatures appear to be able to work to open themselves, allow the flow in a conscious willingness, to give up the little me, but allow "IT" to flow and express and move as you. Maybe "IT" is just having fun, going through all the various awakenings to find itself again, to experience those times when the ego releases and there is freedom. Home while incarnate – something like that.

And maybe, it is simply another level, part of the human potential, this other flow and ease level. After all, the functions of most of our DNA are not understood and I dare say, some we are not yet even aware of.

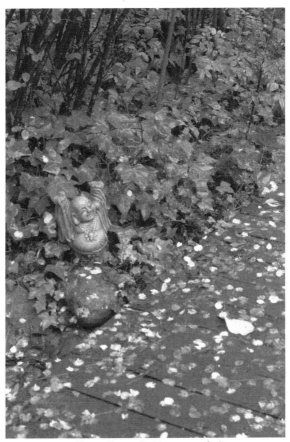

May all walk with Ease and Grace.

"There is also a lot of misery out there
yet YOU can become so spiritualized
that you can actually
do something about the pain

Yes You

but not "you trapped in the robot mind" –
you can't
and not enslaved by human desires and
emotions you won't."

~ E.J. Gold

Can I do Healings For Others?

Yes you can, even untrained.

How?

Listen, listen to the other, listen to what is needed. Be present. Just be there. Don't judge. For distance energy healings, when someone is asking for help, healing thoughts and/or prayers, for him/herself or another, you can go to your place of peace, internally or externally, where your everyday thoughts and worries are let go, and hold the other with compassion in your mind and heart. You can visualize the person or situation in light, or simply wish for the best outcome. You can also channel energy through your hands. Know that the energy will just go where it is needed most. In general, you don't specify for a particular outcome. Just holding him/her in the light. The best outcome is always that in the highest interest of the being of the other, and at least I don't assume to know what that looks like.

You can simply pray for another.

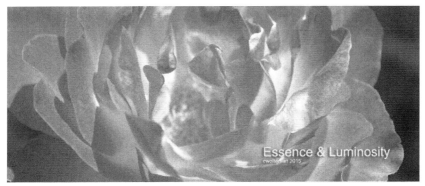

You take yourself out of the equation in terms of what you want for yourself.

For anymore specific healing, you either need to be guided, or learn it somewhere. There are ways to take on someone's energy, but this is ill advised unless you know how to deal with it. The 100% concentration and staying in a certain space until all the dark is transformed is not to be taken lightly. You don't want it to get stuck in your own field somewhere.

If you are grounded into the Earth, you can channel energy from the Earth through your hands into the energy body of another, and allow the dark to be flushed out and to be absorbed by the earth, creating a cycle. This way you don't have to deal with it yourself. The earth is a great and willing healer.

"Conscious believing is the active act of deciding to believe that something is possible such as an unexplained way that an apparently magical effect could have been achieved."

~ E.J. Gold

Snapshot of a Moment on my Journey

Time To Relax

So maybe in the midst of not getting much done, there is a rambling of sorts about – nothing at all.

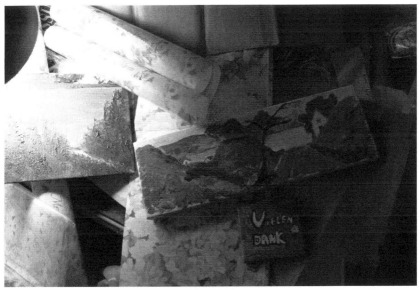

The Gift

Not knowing where I am or where to be in this time where everything seems to be all at once, renders me almost unable to do anything in the midst of projects piled up way above my head. Standing Rock and all those with that purpose, child labor and trafficking, the Russians and

Chinese and the mess in Europe and the Middle East, the microbiome and genetic engineering still in infancy, and what of the oceans and animals everywhere... I could go on and on and on, including the acts of kindness and animal saving and restoration in the face of overwhelming odds against...
Black holes, and gravity and all the ancient myths and miracles and times, mushrooms and poop-eating dogs, hawks eating a sweet chicken I was not able to protect, forever sitting on my lap with her soft feathers that I am stroking, forever running and trying to get away from the hawk who needed to eat, someone's dog dying likely of poison, but they will never know because... they could not afford vet care nor an autopsy, so many lives everywhere and... so many events and it is all always happening now, all of it, and my mind can't grasp it.

No wonder we come back to the simple things.

The breath, this sitting here typing, this guitar playing soft sounds.

There were times in my life I had direction, focus, energy, purpose. Now it is all uncertain.

Transitioning, but no idea into what... holding on to some semblance of functionality... at least those chickens need to be cared for, meals to be prepared.

It feels like my insides are empty as space with vast galaxies while this heart keeps beating. I remember Tom Brown's teachings.

I am no genius, but that does not mean I can't go insane – except there is nothing there.

There is nothing I can do, there is nothing to be done, it happens according to some unwritten code.
My brother wrote today, I feel always connected to him.

Even those ideas of Love and family are no different, just part of the labyrinth through the stillness. This body needs care. This body is hurting, but then, it has been worse.

Sensing weird-seeming things inside. Something inside me keeps coming back to this feeling of peace, as I am doing what I am supposed to do, all the while missing some aspects of what is called Life, and walking with horses. But I do smell the rain and taste the nectar of the Gods which, as its main ingredient, contains quince juice, warm quince juice with some honey and coconut bliss – nectar of the Gods who would have ever guessed that this fruit was so divine. Silence and uncertainty, but I am getting my paperwork together, imagining that it will be less burdensome for those still here when this vessel has ceased to be inhabited by that mysterious thing we call life.

I have no painting days, but there is gardening and something to be done all year long. Maybe there needs to be gardening days and images of the beauty, and maybe I do need that new camera I keep thinking about, for the close-up shots, the clarity, to get better focus for one reason only: to show the beauty that surrounds us in any place, anywhere, in all things.

In the end, I don't want to hurt anyone, even if part of me does, I do want to feel that kind hand on my face, grateful for the laughter and jokes and art and music in my life. There might be two young cats coming to live here, I wonder how that will change things.

Relaxing into it – for in truth, there is nothing else I can do that doesn't lead to more pain.

I have to get up so early tomorrow, this will need to end. My neck and back are looking forward to the evening routine on the floor. Tomorrow may or may not ever come for me, but still, there is food for the chickens in the feed storage this evening, and they will be eating well, thanks to help today. Where is this longing coming from to just sit and breathe… feeling the universes inside the stillness?

All is blessed, all is suffering.

*"'Say hello to the jewel inside the lotus',
meaning bow to the Inner Spirit residing
invisibly in the organic form of the living thing
before you."*

~ E.J. Gold

The Shit

Yes, here it is. The shit. In this case, cow shit. Pardon me – cow dung, cow patty, meadow muffin, cow manure. But there is bull shit, too. Look closely, it is actually providing fertile ground and energy for new growth. It contains the seeds for something new to emerge. And so it is with your shit, your etheric shit. And sometimes, you are full of it. But – look closely. Do you see the new life that comes from it? All that energy in that shit.

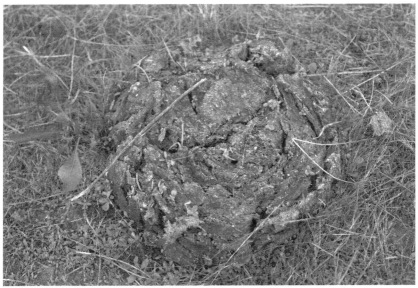

Cow pat and new life

When on the healing journey, and in order for healing – becoming whole – to happen, you will have to face your "stuff", you will have to "own" your dark side, the part of you hidden from plain view. Some call it your "shadow", the part hidden from your everyday consciousness, internal structures, habits and beliefs you are not even aware of. We all have them. Incarnating here is a shock to our Being, a confinement, but nonetheless, as children, our essences shine brightly. Then the family programs get installed, I mean, infants and children are like sponges and absorb and believe everything, belief systems, behavior, attitudes, emotional flavors. For this reason, it is beneficial to expose children to multiple ways of being, languages, music. Life stuff happens, trauma, accidents, abuses of various kinds, cultural norms and rules and expectations, religious indoctrination, and sooner or later, you build a persona, a fake self. You ally with entities, you find a way to shield as much of that vulnerable self as you can, and be able to somehow function in this world. Energy is no longer flowing freely and blocks and distortions ensue. Some things that happen to you get delegated into your unconscious, some things you decide were not so bad and, in fact, okay. Either way, you will need to free yourself of the impact of a lot of that, at least to some degree.

Others can be great mirrors for you. Others can help you see your "stuff", when you are blind to it.

Do you have to relive it all? No. There are trauma therapies and energy therapies and hypnosis these days that allow you to free the trapped energy without getting re-traumatized. There are ways to reprogram yourself without reliving the trauma that made certain habits and beliefs seem acceptable and useful.

You will need to own your shit. Some systems call it shadow work. Often, you yourself are completely unable to see it and it is others who can help you with that. When you get upset about someone else being such and such, or doing this and that, and how bad, unfair, etc. it is – pause, find where it is a reflection of what YOU are being and doing. Putting your shit out there by way of pointing fingers to others is projecting it onto others. I always found it helpful to look at it this way: if you get suddenly upset or something just gets under your skin, chances are you got that same shit running unconsciously, or at the very least, have some unconscious program running that got triggered. If you can look at the other's behaviors calmly, with compassion, if you are simply seeing it, chances are it is theirs. In that case, you need to decide how you would like to live and how you would best deal with it. Sometimes the company you keep is not the company you need to heal.

Sometimes consistently responding differently to a situation will have as a result that over time, the other party also changes. Sometimes you part company.

The other thing that happens a lot is this: you have internal energy and belief structures embedded in your psyche. They got there from your childhood exposures and experiences. If someone or some interaction in your life "triggers" those structures, pathways or feelings, you stop seeing the actual person or situation, but get automatically transported back there... back when it all happened, and sometimes you can't even tell what the hell happened to you. You have transferred something from the past to a present day situation and person. You literally stop seeing the person in front of you and they or the situation, unconsciously, become that person or situation from the past. There is an automatic program running.

One clue that a program was triggered is that later, once it is all over and you look at the situation – and maybe even ask the other person about it – that when you look at it, you see it actually was a pretty small thing. The current situation most often did not at all warrant THAT kind of response. Basically, a neural pathway got triggered through something, could even be something as small as someone walking by wearing a red shirt, and you ran on old automatic circuitry. A reaction not appropriate to the situation is a big clue.

On a healing path, you won't be able to avoid self-observation, examining yourself and your intention.

One question you can ask yourself of any situation: What am I getting out of it?

It helps to know that all these mechanisms – and everyone has conditioning of some kind – happened because you wanted to survive. They are defense mechanisms against getting hurt. However, they eventually stand in the way of you becoming and manifesting as the being you are. They will prevent you from living your highest potential.

Releasing energy blocks and clearing pathways often leads to much more available energy flowing through the system and a new vibrant phase and growth ensues. The energy is no longer held and stuck, but becomes available. This feels great, usually. You need to tend to the pathway, keep it clear so energy does not get stuck there again, which is the tendency. On the path you might find that you revisit the same issues. Something you thought you dealt with back then, resurfaces on a deeper level. Eventually, some things get cleared, while some very very deep structures seem to persist. Some of those structures simply differentiate your incarnation from all others – your "type" is simply different. And that is okay. Even then, meta-programming can also be changed. We are able to express differently. We become fluid.

It is very good for children to be exposed to various types of people, it will help them to remain flexible in how they can express their energy.

In order for the energy to flow freely through you, you need to get more and more clear. On that path, there will be stages, or, to speak with gamer language, levels. You conquer something and level up. Final act boss monsters usually present a special challenge for which you need the tools to handle it.

And here is something I learned from Tom Brown Jr.: When you reach higher levels of being work, there are demons that will take notice, energy beings or entities trying to throw things your way that will make you go back where you came from – a lower level. So far I have found it to be true. There is a different level of "stuff" that happens.

Your intention, determination, ingenuity and power will be called upon, your love for your path, your self, whatever you call it. Don't be afraid to ask for help.

And remember, there are levels of light where the dark no longer has any foothold.

I am just saying this because, at least for me, it has not been steady progress. There were many struggles and setbacks, and it is still not over. Leveling up also does not seem to happen as fast anymore and there appear to be long periods of "no developments" as far as you can see. Those plateaus are to be expected. That is okay, maybe you need to gather energies, fortify your new structures and maybe the great Being, the great Spirit knows when you are ready to move ahead better than you do.

Some people have a defining experience after which their life changes. Some come quite apart and it takes time and work and care to reassemble and become functional again.

Something they taught at the BBSH, and elsewhere, is: Your particular path and struggle is what your soul needs and took on to face and heal to express your greatest gift and service to the all, whatever that is.

Some would seem to come in with a monumental task, others seem to have it "easy". Don't judge it, don't compare it.

You may recall this song:

Row row row your boat

Gently down the stream

Merrily merrily merrily merrily

Life is but a dream

Row row row your boat: Row YOUR boat, not someone else's, take responsibility for you, your actions and the way you live.

Down the stream: go with the flow, not against it, and do it gently, not frantically, upset, grasping. Enjoy what comes your way, enjoy the scenery, but don't paddle back to hold on to it.

Merrily merrily – yes, not frowning or angry… put a smile on your face, laugh.

Life is but a dream – the manifest, now also discovered by quantum mechanics – is not really there… it is a dream. You come in and out of existence constantly. This one is the most difficult to grasp.

One more thing. The shadow is kind of a better way to describe what is unconscious to you, because, what lies in the shadow is not only your shitty stuff and qualities, but also the divine, high-vibrational aspects you may project onto others. Any time you put someone on a pedestal, you are likely projecting something onto them that is one or more of your qualities. It is also very unfair to them to have to live up to that, in fact, they can't and won't – and sometimes they will turn against you, but most of all, it is not serving you.

Point being, sometimes it is harder to own your greatness, your talents, your loving-kindness… simply because it hurts to get those deeply crushed.

When you get punished for being bad, at least that is understandable.

But when you get "punished" for your brilliance, kindness, when your creativity gets squished... that is devastating in a different way, and soon enough, you bury it where no one can ever hurt it again... but you still see it, in others...

It might just be time to own that, too. In order to do your job you came to do in this life, it will be a necessity.

Whenever you are transforming something in yourself, you have done so for everyone in the field who resonates, who faces similar issues. You raise the frequency of the whole... and everyone working in that way contributes to YOUR progress, healing and awakening, too.

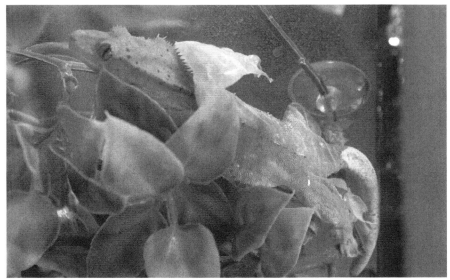

Gecko shedding skin that no longer fits

Are you willing to let go of your old structures, habits and beliefs, which no longer serve your growing, expanding being? Like that gecko's skin – that skin was not bad, it was vital at some point. The skin that no longer serves is shed when the pressure is big enough. May you, too, be able to let go of everything and anything that no longer serves your highest goal and soul's purpose.

The List

This is a list of activities and qualities that help in healing and integration. Simple, everyday things, anyone can do them. No need to do them all, not all at once anyway. You will find the ones that work best for you. Is this list complete? Hell no, there is so much more, but ya gotta start somewhere.

- Exercise
- Learn mindfulness
- Connect with the earth, be in nature

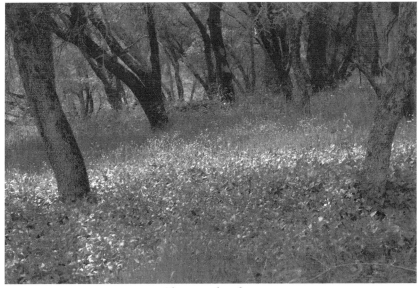

She can heal us

- Pick any practice and do it for 5 minutes each day (as in play guitar, sit and pay attention to your breathing, do a drawing...)
- Nourish your body and mind with real food, real food which supports your body-healing and mental wellness, not poisons it
- Meditation (if not disassociating)
- Sit down and feel what is going on in your body
- State your perspective on something, then take a different perspective, then find another perspective on the same issue, then another one
- Good people around you
- Observe surroundings
- Notice your feelings, observe your reaction, observe your thoughts
- Observe your thoughts and how they make you feel. Try a different thought and notice how that makes you feel
- Self-honesty
- Be kind and gentle with yourself
- Journaling & writing
- Drawing
- Painting
- Singing
- Danceing
- Make music, play/learn an instrument
- Volunteering
- No cell phone and no internet time
- Spending time with family and friends
- Create community
- Rest when needed
- Communicate what must be communicated
- Find what you love to do, what you are passionate about
- Discover your life's purpose
- Get out of the box, try something new
- Become flexible
- Learn new things, investigate and research
- Develop a sense of humor, laugh at yourself and lighten up.
- Connect – with your self, your family, your community, with animals

- Sit opposite someone and gaze into their eyes for a few minutes, dogs count and may be easier for some (or many)
- Find beauty, wherever you live
- Practice gratitude
- Be kind to someone
- Smile more
- When constantly thinking the same thoughts… DO something unrelated
- Play
- Do "nothing"
- Play Move-Act Code
- Seek professional help when needed

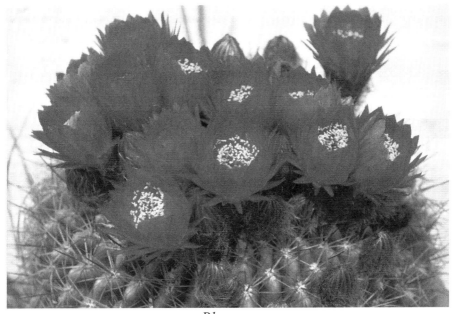

Blossom

Breathe and Move
Be Kind to Yourself
Always Remember Gratitude

Here are a few programs, work, people and methods to check out that I can personally recommend: Tom Brown Jr, the Tracker School, Hakomi, BBSH, Pathwork, The Work of Byron Katie, Waking Down in Mutuality, Core Energetics, Reiki, Matrixworks with Mukara Meredith, Tools of Transformation at IDHHB with E.J. Gold, Integral Practice, Eckhart Tolle, Cameli and Arjuna Ardagh, Family Constellation (Hellinger), Reiki, Thomas Hübl, Natural Dog Training (Kevin Behan), Diane Musho Hamilton, Emotional Freedom Technique, Yoga, Dancing, Pottery, CranioSacral Therapy, work with animals. There are many more methods and books, too numerous to count.

"If you don't like something, change it. If you can't change it, change your attitude."

~ Maya Angelou

"You can't change what it is, you can see it, you can learn from it, but you can't change it."

~ E.J. Gold

Odds and Ends

Honestly, there were just a couple more quotes that wanted to be in this book, and a little story involving my mother, which prompted me to write a little about stages of human development.

A couple of weeks ago I was on the phone with my mom in Germany. Religion came up, as it usually does. This time she said something like: "...that is not looking good, it looks pretty dark, I might be losing my faith." On the other hand, she still clings to Jesus being the only one, and says she is too old to learn something new, she does not want that new stuff (she is 80). We have often discussed that the values: love, help, be kind, etc, are really universal, everywhere, even in other religions. Even Jesus was kind to the "others"... still, she clings to Jesus as being THE son of God and through him salvation is to be had. Yet, she is in a crisis, and this is a sign that she is growing. At the same time, resisting change most definitely.

Humans go through developmental stages of growing up. This happens in several areas, or lines, of development, like moral, spiritual/religious, thinking/cognitive. To give a simplified example of what is meant by developmental stages, let us use the example of the development of caring.

At the early stage of development, stage 1, there is ME, it's all about me.

The stage is also called egocentric, selfish, narcissistic and someone at this stage is unable to take the role of others. It is all about Me.

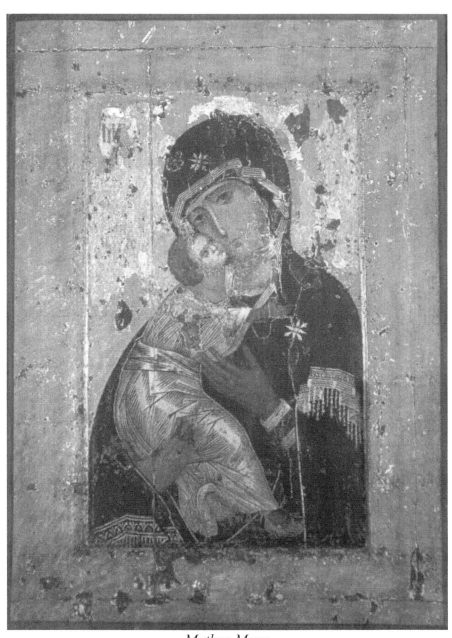

Mother Mary

At stage 2, care develops from me to us. Care extends to a group. It is us vs. them. People at this stage are group-centric. This stage gives rise to racists, sexists, homophobia. Religious fundamentalism, the one and only true path, is at this stage.

At stage 3, care develops towards all humans, we call it world-centric and one tends to (wants to) treat all people fairly.

At stage 4, care extends to all beings. Masculine and feminine are integrated, identity and moral care expands to all beings, the integral stage is cosmo-centric.

Every major study of love has shown that it expands and increases with every major level of development, from selfish me-only love, to small group love, to large group love, to love of all humanity to love of all beings.

"In other words, evolution and love go hand in hand, an example of spirit in action if ever there was one. The more we love, the more we flourish. The more morally sensitive we are, the wider our own circle of identity goes from an isolated me to all sentient beings, and then the universe itself in total, a supreme identity with the ground of all being."

~ Ken Wilber

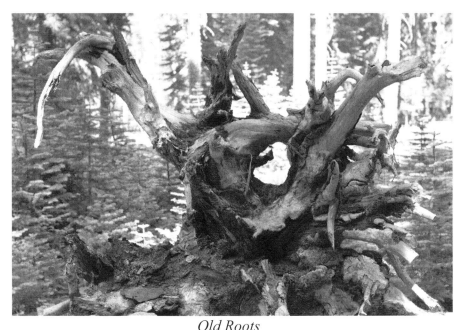

Old Roots

photo courtesy of Helena from The Living Sculptures

So what does that look like for someone her/his losing her faith?

Let us say someone of the Christian faith has a true waking experience, a divine light experience, ultimate love experience, the ultimate unity experience with the light being – Jesus Christ.

At Stage 1 of religious/spiritual development, you will think you are Jesus Christ.

Waking up is full, growing up is at the lowest level, the "me me me" – level. And yes, you are Jesus Christ, so is everyone else with that same experience. For someone at Stage 1 to acknowledge that others can claim the same is impossible.

At Stage 2 you will think this experience of religious unity is the savior of your special group and this experience of religious unity, Jesus is the personal savior and only chosen people can have this experience. One must accept Jesus as personal savior. You experience oneness, but only your people enjoy that. Your duty: convince or coerce non-believers. Jihad, crusades come with this stage.

This is where large parts of the world population currently sit. The process into the next stage, Stage 3 is difficult and can be experienced as losing one's faith,

However, even Catholic church acknowledges that salvation is possible in other religions.

It is one of the most important transformations, going from Stage 2 to Stage 3 of religious development.

At Stage 3 you will start to see Jesus not as one and only, but as one of several world teachers. It is a difficult step to take for many.

All that to give you a glimpse of this: profound awakening experiences can happen to humans at any stage of development and it can be a totally genuine experience. Now comes the thing, though: even though a true enlightened unity experience happened, if the "growing up" stage is low, then that experience will be interpreted according to the stage of religious development someone is at, or to quote Ken Wilber:

"...we will interpret that waking up state according to the stage of growing up we are at ..."

~ Ken Wilber

Going from one stage to another has often been tumultuous for me. It often feels like dying, transitioning. However, after having gone through the tunnel, really new insights and vistas open up and you can look back at the way you used to be. It is quite fascinating.

Hang in there, and take care of your body and being as best you can in the process.

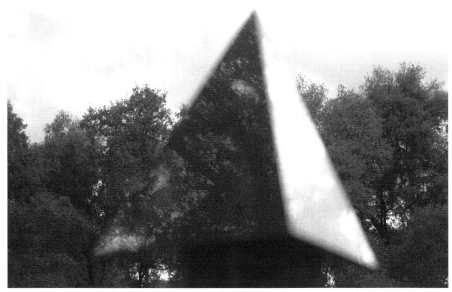

Tetrahedron – Copper Sculpture by Jim Rodney

"If you want others to be happy, practice compassion. If you want to be happy, practice compassion."

~ His Holiness the 14th Dalai Lama

Epigenetics looks at changes in people and their offspring following environmental stresses. A person's experience as a child or teenager can have a profound impact on their future children's lives, including the levels of hormones and how they are processed. What your parents experienced does have consequences in your physiology.

Another important point I wanted to remind you of: An organism's growth is not possible if it is on protection mode. In a state of fear, the organism is in protection mode.

"The most important growth promoting signal for a human is Love."

~ Dr. Bruce Lipton

It is your filters, your perception of your environment, which controls your behavior. If you change your filters, your conditioning, your environment literally will change your gene expression and your behavior. Your perception of the environment rewrites your genes, your active genes. When you give up a belief and change your behavior, your biochemical self changes concurrently. It is not really news, but new enough that it has not made it into any textbooks.

You might have heard many times that it is important to uncover and change your beliefs. You perceive according to your belief and belief changes your genes. It really makes it all the more important to look at your beliefs and change them. Who you are will literally change.

Isn't it it neat that biochemically, we change according to beliefs and environmental stimuli? Our biochemistry changes according to our environment, and our perceived environment depends on our filters and beliefs.

What keeps you in balance is clear perception.

You might have noticed that I am repeating the importance of gratitude. First of all, I have experience with the practice, based on something I read. The feeling of gratitude changes who you are. When one takes findings in recent years into consideration, gratitude changes your perception of your life, and you literally (including biochemically and genetically) change. I think that is such a beautiful supporting little fact.

In my own process and realization, I have come to this: Love is always there, Love IS, and it is always accessible, and ultimately, you are Love. It is always there and you are never separate from it. I know, I had heard it many times, but once you actually experience the truth of it, it is a different ballgame. It is up to us to recognize it. It is important to dismantle our old limiting beliefs, patterning, filters, and give our body and mind and soul an environment where it feels safe, give it food and impressions and practices to grow and expand. Self-observation and shadow work is good to illuminate your beliefs and blinders. Being gentle and kind to yourself is important.

One of the functions of our healing space is this: to be a container to allow relaxation with the intention for healing. Relax and open and let the energy flow through you. Allow visions, subtle states of being, going into deep peace and emptiness, but cling to none.

Already it is in the field, in line with the importance of daily practice, to investigate doing a daily transmission to set the tone of the day, like a mini meditation, setting intention. It already feels like it needs to happen, however, this does stretch my technical abilities.

I was listening this afternoon to the archive of the Saturday morning talk of the Labor Day Convention 2017 of IDHHB. Here are some points made by E.J. Gold, some of which happen to be resonating with this topic.

Transcribed:

"Regarding the current environment: Survival has to do with a number of factors: Humor, marketing, good sense, good values and an ability to tread the right path.

"When you are acting under divine guidance, you can't go wrong.

"The bottom line for everything, all of existence, is: How are you spending your time and with whom? It's about your company and right action.

"You have a job, which is to prepare yourself for the next level of existence, the next level of work, the next level of life. You move on by moving on, by rising, by transcending… it's an alchemical process.

"Attunement has to do with changing the vibration of yourself, of your SELF, the whole thing, changing the atomic vibration of yourself. You can do that with meditation, yes, that is one way. Your other practices that will work to some degree as well, they all work to some degree, some greater or lesser degree… depending on you, the situation and circumstances, how well the system that you are using fits you at this time…

"Your understanding is very important. That comes from compassion, mostly from compassion, from seeing other points of view…

"Vegetarian is not in itself more spiritual than some other form of ingestion and processing food. However, it is more conscious, it is more considered, it is kinder. Your body will tell you if it wants to be fed certain foods. If it does not want those foods and you force those foods on the body, you find that you have to flavor those foods for the body to accept it.

"You are here to do a little work, to do some work.

"It is time, place and people. One of the skills that you need to develop is a way of actually reinventing your work and the work of the people around you.

"The world is changing very radically, very rapidly.

"And as the world changes, it will have radical significance to you because there will be times and places where you will not be permitted to do this work openly.

"I am taking the alchemical process which is a growth process, an evolutionary process and moving it into kind of one-on-one… engineering it onto the POD process…"

Much later during that morning, paraphrased: "When you produce (this stone, this philosopher's stone), the process you go through to make that happen is gonna change everything… change the vibration not just of your body, but of your very being. That is the function of the alchemical process."

"Right action is always guided by conscience and consciousness."

~ E.J. Gold

The Cats

In 1987, 30 years ago, I adopted two kittens from a kill shelter in Baltimore. I had to have two because as a medical resident, every third night I would not be home, doing 36-hour shifts. I played with them, I loved them and I cared for them the way most people do: commercial food, litter boxes, some toys. They moved with me, first to New York, then back to Germany for two years, then back to the United States where we moved three times again. One, the hunter of the two, died of an embolus due to an unknown heart disease at age 8. The other one cried so much she lost her voice. At that time, I realized that there was something there I didn't really understand about cats. As if they had types of feelings I didn't know they had. And it is not that they were still as close as they had been the first two years. During one of the moves, I had to leave one behind for two months, after which time they never again slept cuddled up or groomed each other. Still, they were always in the same house or apartment, and obviously the one left behind missed her? The remaining cat was a great helper when I moved in with a housemate and friend, who later got diagnosed with cancer. She stopped working and the cat kept her company, for years.

When I moved to California, the remaining cat was 16, she had gotten used to my coming and going and frequent staying away for a week or two over the years. So when I said goodbye this time, for her it was no different. She stayed with my friend, but later lived with our neighbors. The cat died about 2 years later. How can I tell? She visited me while I was sleeping, the only such time. I heard her purr and could feel her weight and paws kneading on my chest so much that I woke up. That was her goodbye.

By that time, I had started helping out in a garden run by someone else. The day before harvesting, we were to let the plants know about it. Though it made sense, I did not actually understand it at the time, but I did it.

Years later, after a major transition, I understand why it is so important to let the plants know ahead of time. There is a big difference in how I sense/experience animals and plants. Yes, I went through an entirely sentimental phase, but at some point I realized, saw, felt that out of any animal's eyes, there is consciousness looking back at you – THE consciousness. The "spirit that moves through all things", animates all things, is the same. It only looks out through different eyes and different forms of being. There is, amidst all the differences, an underlying spirit, soul, beingness, a consciousness, that is the same. And it does not stop at sentient animals, and then with plants, any plant, all plants. Are there any non-sentient creatures? My edge are the inanimate "things", inert things, I can see how one could sense the same spirit in atoms and molecules, but, I can't – yet.

"The mineral world is a much more supple and mobile world than could be imagined by the science of the ancients. Vaguely analogous to the metamorphoses of living creatures, there occurs in the most solid rocks, as we now know, perpetual transformation of a mineral species."

~ Pierre Teilhard de Chardin

But can you imagine how much more pain there suddenly is when you realize the nature of other sentient beings, animals and plants, ecosystems included? Actually, if you are not there yet, you can't even imagine it. I never "thought" that abusing animals was right, or destroying forests, but I didn't feel it the same way as now.

Back to the cat story. I can remember how it was with my first cats, and then – there was Tiny Lacy. I have written in detail about my adventure with adopting two feral cats at helpingk9s.com.

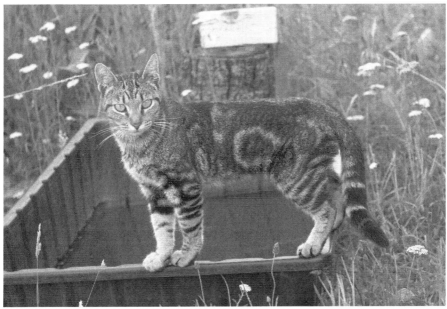
Tiny Lacy

Tiny Lacy came to me as one of two recently caught and neutered young, about 9 months old, feral cats in December, 2016. I didn't see her for days as she was hiding in the box that I put in the crate used during the relocation process. She was the shy one of the two. Over seven months, the transformation was amazing. Being free garden cats, I am floored at her beingness, her trusting, her sensitivity, gentleness, yielding, attention. She did hunt the gophers, too.

Certain aspects of her qualities became super apparent after a distance healing I did with her in the morning of July 7th - because she had just about stopped eating and was getting so thin (not a new thing, just seemed worse). She ate more that afternoon after the healing than the three days before that. I remedied one distress factor, another feral cat and her kittens that had shown up during the winter and that I was taking care of. And I also kept her vet appointment that same day, where she was diagnosed with feline leukemia.

She ate well for the next ten days. She put on some weight, her energy came back and I had fantasies of her being able to beat the feline leukemia. Being a garden cat, I saw her about three times a day.

She became super affectionate, seeking eye contact, melting and yielding on my lap under my hands.

The last time she sat, or rather laid, on my lap (before this hunter became the hunted and got killed by dogs, having ventured out of the safe garden area), there was a space between us that was – as if substantial, like a very very very fine plasma. It was divine, this feeling of profound and mutual connection, of love. She slightly turned her head and glanced back at me. There was a lover energy sense about this gesture and moment. It was out of this world. It caught me a bit by surprise, but I remember the moment it happened. I even noticed a questioning in my mind "LOVE, is that possible with a cat?" The big Love-Space. The You and Me Love-Space. What exactly is this? I still can't place it. I know there is consciousness everywhere, including in animals, but this was just extraordinary.

And I am recalling as I am writing that at age 29 I declared the meaning of my life be: to learn to love, the big Love. Unlimited Love. I wondered about Love since the age of 12, walking next to my aunt, pushing a baby carrier. I came to the conclusion that since I was willing to give my arm so that my baby niece could live, that had to be love.

I miss Tiny cat. She was a delight to me every time I went into the garden. That momentary space we shared was truly remarkable, standing out from all others. At the same time, I am at peace and grateful, so grateful for this experience.

When I look at the events of the day, when Tiny Lacy left, I can see the various influences and conditions that lead to the experiences we each had and those we shared, and her death. I can say: If I had done such and such, she would have likely lived longer, but no one knows if that would have been better. She did have feline leukemia, and she was an outdoor cat. And there were other cats that showed up who needed care. So who is to know what would have been "better"? We reached a space that was amazing, and while I have experienced remarkable spaces, this one had a different flavor to it. It fits somewhere on the spectrum of what is possible, but I am not educated enough to place it.

I trust in Being, and maybe the mission of her life in the grander scheme of things is being fulfilled by me writing about her in this book calling for healing. I delighted in her presence, the way she was, ran, jumped, looked at me, shot past me on the garden paths. She is missed. But now, after about a month, there is pretty much just gratitude and a sense of peaceful, deep, quiet joy.

This human, me, came to love her, or rather, experience a love space in a way that is new to me. I was not able to love my other cats 30 years ago, in this way. And I am telling you: growing up, becoming more and more whole, is worth it. I recall the German shepherd-husky, Skye, which I took care of for seven months a few years ago and had remarkable experiences with. Both experiences have in common these things or attitudes, which are: saying 100% yes to providing and taking care of the animal, which included observing them, studying them, connecting with them, sacrificing for them, spending time with them, sitting with them, modifying what was needed for them, allowing them to give their trust, on their own terms and in their own time.

One might argue that it was a special cat, and I don't deny that just as there are differences in the ability and developments in humans, that such differences also might exist in animals. Maybe it was just a vibratory compatibility and resonance. In any case, I simply would not have been able to recognize it, to vibrate like that, 30 years ago. I wasn't there yet. Maybe in order for this special moment of divine-love-space-substance to be there, it took both a special cat and my ability to sense it. Some animals come into our lives to help raise our consciousness. She was one of those.

"Love alone is capable of uniting living beings in such a way as to complete and fulfill them, for it alone takes them and joins them by what is deepest in themselves."

~ Pierre Teilhard de Chardin

One of the points that I am trying to make is: 30 years ago, the kind of experience I had with Tiny Lacy was not likely to happen. In fact, it possibly could not happen because of where I was at internally at the time. Equally, I don't know how an experience with another cat in the future might be if I grow and expand more.

So many factors contributed to her life ending when it did, I can see the interconnectedness of events far beyond my direct involvement. Because the connection was experienced as something so exquisite and extraordinary, I am writing about it for you – for you to hear that 30 years ago, who I was and what I was open to and able to do and experience, I would have not been able to feel/sense it the same way. There was nothing wrong with how I was with my first cats, I did love them dearly and gave them a good life. But this is a different level.

Her death seems premature to me, but on the other hand, she is making it just in time to be included in this book for you to hear about this and consider that growing and evolving, even with the growing pains it brings, is worth it. As it concerns loving, you are able to love, sense love and be love in ways that you didn't before, and could not even imagine.

"The deep pain that is felt at the death of every friendly soul arises from the feeling that there is in every individual something which is inexpressible, peculiar to him alone, and is, therefore, absolutely and irretrievably lost."

~ Arthur Schoppenhauer

The above quote spoke to me when losing some of the chickens living in that same garden. I am no longer sure about the validity of the last part of that quote. I agree that there was something unique about this cat that cannot ever be repeated. But, there is a component of what happened in the exchange, that recognition of another as Love, that at this time I believe does stay with Being forever. It is not all lost. It changes "IT", that which IS, forever. It fulfilled a purpose. It was done, and Being – that which IS – is changed as well as nourished through it. I can't prove it, I can't really explain it. It is not the first time events came together for me to get this sense. There is something about a true love-trust-space that can be experienced by us at a level where there are no words and it is not limited to human-human interactions, and it is not ever lost. It was exquisitely beautiful and felt real.

Love is like that, it wants the connection, the wholeness in this manifest reality. I don't even know that it is limited to sentient beings, but hey, the journey continues.

This moment was an indication, an inkling of the lover relationship one can develop with the Absolute in the form of creation.

Sometimes when evolving, growing and transforming on our healing journey, the going gets excruciatingly tough. Sometimes things look pretty dark inside and out, sometimes you almost fall apart and that is all part of the process. Growing pains can be difficult. Hang in there. It's worth it. Remember self care in the process. Be kind to yourself!

My experience with this cat, "Tiny", includes one of those eternal moments that will stay with me. Even though I have no way of proving it, this experience with her did something to Being itself – it changed "IT" and it is now different. Maybe it simply fulfilled something.

Just a short note on "Life". Life IS. The way I see it, Life is part of what IS and will always, in any manifest world, assert itself. It pushes on. Development happens, and just like there are various levels of development in humans, so are there different levels of individual animals within a species. As a whole, animals, too, are evolving, which is just the Latin word for developing. That is simply part of the nature of Life in the Kosmos.

In your healing journey, the journey of becoming whole and realizing who you are, you will end up feeling so much more. It starts with feeling and accepting any rejected, previously disowned and hidden parts of yourself, but then, if you continue, you will become more and more aware and sensitive to all kinds of living beings and situations. It will not be all joy and bliss. It will also mean that you will feel more pain, a LOT more pain. At the same time, it is all as it should be and unfolding as it is according to a blueprint and plan that is not rooted in your individual consciousness. It is humbling, in a good way. There is more compassion for yourself and all living beings, all of creation. You might find that you care for it all more, wanting to be of the highest service you can be, to the best of your ability and circumstance. It is good. It is beautiful.

"You need this love to be grounded, until there is no difference between you and your love, or what you love or what you are. It's just the one thing."

~ Leonard Cohen

"Love is an adventure and a conquest. It survives and develops, like the universe itself, only by perpetual discovery."

~ Pierre Teilhard de Chardin

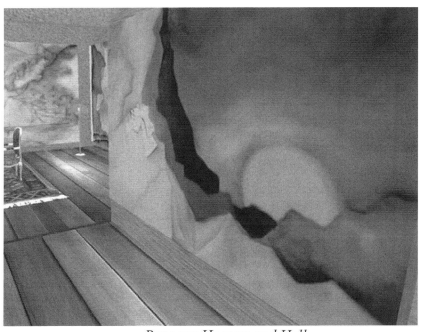

Between Heaven and Hell

Prosperity Virtual Ashram

Art by E.J. Gold

Original oil on 5x7 ft canvas

"If by eternity is understood not endless temporal duration but timelessness, then he lives eternally who lives in the present."

~ Ludwig Wittgenstein

DEH Notes

DEH stands for Distance Energy Healing. After each healing event, I write down some notes and post them online for the week in case participants wish to compare notes or want to know more. Sometimes there are messages to share.

We only started recently, therefore, the small number of notes.

I have gotten some encouraging and unsolicited feedback and comments about the effect of the healing work from people who have attended the events. It feels good that this is helpful and I am grateful they were willing to share. Here is the website where the notes are posted, usually within 24 hours of the event. They will be available for one week, till the next healing event.
http://www.let-the-healing-begin.com/

*"I live in Heaven.
I work in Hell."*

~ E.J. Gold

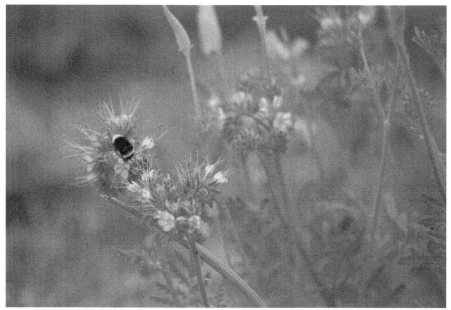

Evening Forager

"The adventure of awakening is among the most universal of human dramas."

~ Ken Wilber
Integral Life Practice: A 21st Century Blueprint for Physical Health,
Emotional Balance, Mental Clarity, and Spiritual Awakening

DEH 01 – Notes from June 9, 2017

This past Friday, on June 9, 2017, we had our first Distance Energy Healing space on GorebaggTV.

There are a couple of reasons to share this, one being that we will have to modify the event description.

The event description needs to reflect that it is okay to be in the space, but specific agreement for individual energy work is needed, indicated by signing in with OCD or speaking YES in your own space once the healing session has begun. For those who know about OCD (originally Open Channel Didge) – it stands for Open Channel DistanceEnergyHealing.

How I came to that conclusion:

A space opened up that was very close to a familiar area from a lucid dream I had years ago. While I didn't see the temple-like building or the lake, it was not far from either, just a short walking distance.

There were many beings in the space, and once the healing began, several light helpers did help a number of them. The entire area was overseen/observed by many spirit guides. I sense hesitation, like a lot of beings there were not sure about asking for energy work. It turns out that even though attendance in the space was considered a request for help, that at least as far as "I" was concerned, I can't just walk up to anyone there and do energy work without specific request… indicated by a stepping forward or a "YES".

At some point, some of the assembled stepped forward for healing energy. Between those times, I was simply holding space and observing.

Of those asking for energy healing, most remained standing, but one especially was lying on a table in front of me. A fairly large, about soccer ball-sized area in what would be corresponding to the upper right abdomen, was shaded, with a black pointy smaller object stuck in it from the median side. This was causing illness in the physical. The task was to either loosen and remove or transform the pointy object. It got loosened up energetically, with the help of two guides, but even they were unable to slowly remove it. It seemed very stuck. So we had to go back and ask: Are you ready to let go of this? And there was hesitation, and basically, when it came down to it, they were not ready.

So other work went on for a while. One little being was just that, little, about 18 inches tall. He was very happy afterward. Later we heard back: Okay, I am ready now. With light and gentle persistence, the pointy "object" got loosened completely from its embeddedness and gently removed, filling the space with light. The two guides pretty much did that.

After this session, it became clear to me that even though many were in the space, only some stepped forward to receive some healing work, and those were the only ones I am permitted to work with directly.

So yes, you can be in the space, but unless you somehow indicate your wish and agreement for healing work to happen, it won't. Not even the guides can do that. You will still receive the general benefit of being in the space and the energy, just not receive any energy work yourself specifically. We will modify the event description.

Did I perceive this vs. making it all up? This is not easy to answer if you have no personal experience of high sense perception. I decided to share one of the most pivotal events in my own life regarding this that can partially answer this question. It involves the Healer Woman soapstone carving you can see on the Healing Altar.

When in a learning space with others, you end up getting enough confirmation along the way that you are not making it up, that you just know. When I am clear, high-sense perception works best and is reliable. I don't walk around like that because I don't want to know and it is none of my business. But in an intentionally provided space, and if needed, high-sense perception kicks in and I have learned to trust it.

DEH – Notes 2 - from June 16-2017

The technical stuff: lag can be really long. After we were done and I got back to my own computer, the music was still on… until 11:45, that is 25 minutes since it finished in the barn. In the future, we will open the space early for folks to type in any questions… but in the end, whenever the music ends for you, take it easy. I also noticed that I did not hear the bell sound at the end. So hopefully we will fix that.

In my post from last week, you can read why I changed the blurb for the event. Anyone is welcome to attend the event and be in the space. If you are open to or wish for specific energy work, this can be indicated by typing OCD (Open Channel DistanceEnergyHealing) in the chat or indicate in your own space – yes, speaking either aloud or telepathically.

As to the healing space-time itself, there is the obligatory grounding and connecting, but as soon as that was done, someone seemed ready. I did a chelation (meaning to charge and balance the energy field). From the start, there seemed a huge light presence in the general assembly space that I did not "see" last week. While there were some guides working with beings, this presence seemed to take over. I could sense but not see past it.

There was some channeling energy with a complete circle from the depth of the inner earth, healer, recipient and back into the Earth. The Earth is a great healer and source of energy, especially for our bodies. If you can find a spot to lie down on bare Earth… do so.

There were other little healings… and the space expanded and expanded. If you were able to go there, you noticed how it felt.

It became clear that the greatest healing lies in the recognition of the truth of reality. From there, manifesting is fluid, not solid. It is your consciousness and intention that is the ultimate healer.

It is equally clear that the space and, indeed, very beingness is shared.

"The ultimate aim of the quest must be neither release nor ecstasy for oneself, but the wisdom and power to serve others."

~ **Joseph Campbell**

DEH – Notes from June 23, 2017

Once the space was open, the first and most obvious thing I noticed was a huge black something coming in from the left and almost covering the field all the way across it and about two-thirds into the back. Several beings attended to it. Slowly it transformed and dispersed.

Someone with a pointy energy almost from head to toe was the first of several receiving energy work. About two-thirds of the way through, the space went pretty high, though not as expanded as last week.

The immense number of humans suffering became obvious as the space expanded to show many who were waiting, lost, ignorant, suffering. Are you ready to let it go? This question came up a couple of times and was shared in the chat.

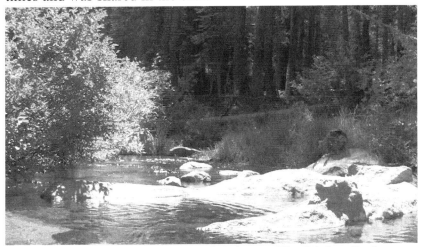

Resting – Image courtesy of Helena – The Living Sculptures

"The recent explosion of interest in alternative care – including such disciplines as psychoneuroimmunology – has made it quite clear that the person's interior states (emotions, psychological attitude, imagery and intentions) play a crucial role in both the cause and the cure of even physical illness."

~Ken Wilber

DEH Notes 4 – June 30, 2017

The space was opened and the area looked to be the same place, but it had changed. The colors were different, certain types of surrounding had disappeared… and though I tried for a moment to just see it like it used to be, it didn't work. Initially, there was movement today in the space by the beings there, almost as if milling about. It took a while to get settled. Remind yourself that this is all on the energy/spirit level.

Initially, a huge, dark, slender shape, many times the size of the people beings, was standing there looking around as if to see who it can attach to or snap up. However, it was firmly told to leave and it just dissolved. Higher energy beings were starting to work. This is all still in the first five minutes. A huge cube appeared hovering above the space, somewhat golden in color. Never seen it before. Then I found myself inside the cube. There were plasma movements and more inside, and then it opened up to infinite space.

This is difficult to describe, but for those who were tuned in, you'll know. We stayed in that space for a long time after that. There were several beings who requested specific energy healing work, and I won't go into that here.

The boundaries of the healing plaza/space were less firm… and there were many, many more beings extending far beyond the original space.

Then the collective grounding phase started, kind of by itself. This was pretty amazing. In this case, it meant that all who were there, to some degree or totally, allowed themselves to be connected deep into the Earth (this was energetic)… at the same time remaining open and connected to the infinite space. THIS is really the space of highest healing potential, however it may manifest individually, which may be different for each person. Do NOT ever discount your own perception of what happened. It is what is right for you. You might have been tuned into a different frequency, your high- sense perception shows the space to you the way YOU perceive it. Maybe you hear it, maybe you see colors much better. Just mentioning this in case any doubt comes up for you.

A couple more specific healings happened, and then I mostly remained in that space, allowing other energy beings to do the work, and allowing everyone to simply experience what is.

To ground down is to connect with the Earth. Not being grounded makes it difficult to fully embody. The task for this week, if you wish to do it, is to stand in your space, feet about shoulder width apart, knees not locked. Gently tilt the pelvis back and forth a few times till you sense the best position. You can put your hands in prayer position or just leave the arms on your sides. Then imagine a line from the top of your head straight down through the center of your pelvis to the molten core of the Earth. Feel your feet on the ground, your energy extending deep into the ground. You can also start the line in the center of your pelvic area, about a couple of inches under the belly button. If you can do this barefoot somewhere, all the better. For those unable to stand, do it sitting up, or, if lying down, you can imagine your body slowly sinking into the ground while energy strands connect you to the center of the Earth. You can take time out in nature and sit somewhere to do this. The Earth itself is a great healer for human bodies.

May all walk in ease and grace. Have a blessed week.

Dok

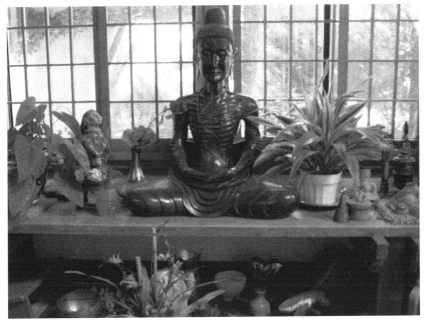

Buddy The Buddha – The Fasting Buddha

"There is no substitute for the triumph of Will."

~ E.J. Gold

"A thought is harmless unless we believe it."

~ Byron Katie

DEH Notes 5 July 7, 2017

It was interesting that the familiar physical surroundings as perceived through high sense-perception appeared almost non-existent. There was mostly light everywhere.

A few animals showed up, too, one of which was a big bear. Several healings were done, which again I will not be specific about except for this message: Go gently. At the end, some high vibrational guides where appearing and seemed to be smiling and/or grinning. That made me smile.

Thank you to those who were there. May all walk with ease and grace.

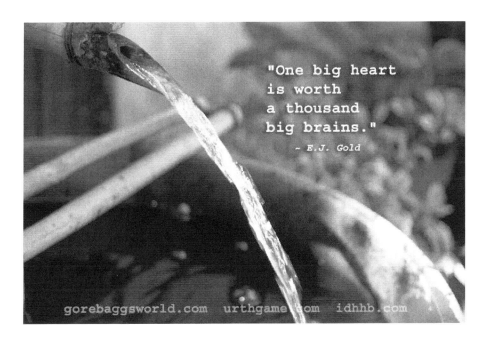

"One big heart
is worth
a thousand
big brains."
~ E.J. Gold

gorebaggsworld.com urthgame.com idhhb.com

"The beauty of practice is that it transforms us so that we outgrow our original intentions— and keep going! Our motivations for practicing evolve as we mature."

~ Ken Wilber

"Communication is a habit, not an option."

~ E.J. Gold

DEH Notes 6, July 14, 2017

Today it took quite some time to get settled. There were some local disruptions, which probably, at least as far as the music was concerned, did not affect the transmission. I basically turned the healing space over to the guides for the first 10 minutes, trusting in the higher vibrations.

The space, in high perception, looked about the same as last week, mostly light – not at all anymore like I used to see it. Guides were working, I did hold the space, and two healings. There was some re-configuring of DNA. We ended up in a very high infinite space, after a period of time of going in and out of it. Somewhere in the middle of the time, there were energetic happenings that reminded me of bardo spaces… remember, these are projections. Towards the end there was a short time of big energy bursts.

I love that high infinite still space. It feels like true home. At the end I asked the guides if there was a message. This seemed to be met with something like a compassionate smile…as in: "humans, they need that – messages." The message is: Be yourself, as in true to yourself. And something else that went with it… which I cannot remember.

"There are no obstructions on the path. Everything is the path, including the obstructions."

~ E.J. Gold

"The truth will not necessarily set you free, but truthfulness will."

~ Ken Wilber,
A Brief History of Everything

DEH – notes from July 21, 2017

The assembly space looked about the same as last week. Again we had technical sound issues locally (not online) and it took a while to get settled. It made me realize a potential issue, a dependency on certain sounds to reach the inner state of the healing space. In any case, a good opportunity to do almost without.

It is good to be able to count on the guides to be there, and I trust them completely. I did a couple of healings that were individual, but mostly one banishing and one transformation. This came about because, whether I wanted it or not, my perspective in relation to the space changed from standing at ground level to hovering above it. This happened somewhere towards the 20-minute mark into the healing. It allowed for perception of a much larger area and surrounding energy, revealing a lot of surrounding darkness, which is always ready to invade, and wanted to invade. So it got pushed back with light rays and leaving no doubt about it – the intention that it was not going to enter. The other time, a different form of dark appeared over the field. The darkness transformed when met with the light.

Earlier on there was a word repeated several times, but I cannot recall it.

At some point after the energy transformation, a lot of what could be described as light equivalents of flower petals were gently "raining" on the space. It was delightful and nourishing.

The message in this one is: You do not have to let the darkness in – it needs your agreement and inattention. You can push it back or transform it, if you stand in your truth, integrity and intention, it cannot invade or take over.

There are pockets of light and healing, and, there is darkness everywhere, too. You can keep the space clear and your own energy bodies clear with intention and awareness.

May you walk with ease and grace – Dok

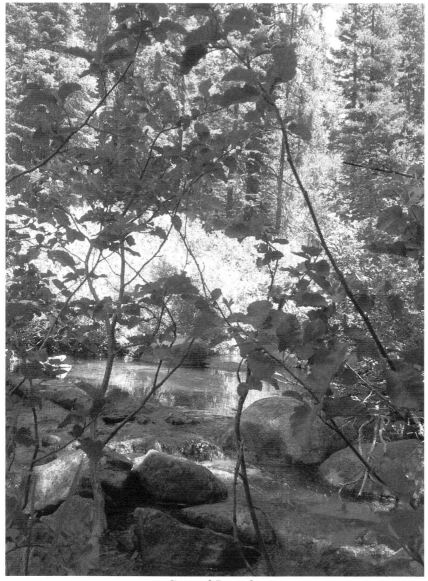

Sacred Breath
Image courtesy of Fred – Blueladder

DEH notes from July 28, 2017

This morning the high perception healing space seemed to have no large or small dark energy blobs in it. It seemed a little bit more colored towards yellowish, golden yellowish light. More colors showed up, spiraling into a funnel/wormhole opening. The funnel then was all around and a little energetically rocky during the passing through the entry to another space, just light and a certain vibratory space. We or I stayed near the entry/exit of the funnel, having gone through it.

There was one healing happening early on, then a charging and balancing in the space some time after passing through the funnel opening. I don't recall everything that happened.

It was interesting to perceive our usual healing space as fully functional with healings happening, sort of "behind" us. This light space was more pure light – willing to infuse the cells of whoever is there with energy for transformation and restructuring. (It got pretty warm/hot for me there). It was pretty amazing to be there.

Do these spaces potentially and/or actually exist at the same "time-space"? Yes. Why they appeared separated I am not sure. I think it might be to help differentiate which type of energy work happens in which space.

Anyway, toward the end of the time in that space, a lot of chakra openings/charging was happening for anyone willing to be there. For some folks the color red in their lives could be important right now. We, or at least I, ended up back in the healing space we have come to know. The transition back was almost without any kind of energetic phenomena. There was no specific message, just the general sense of availability of transformational energy, if you give yourself the time and space to actually be there.

"There's nothing like experience to teach wisdom."

~ E.J. Gold

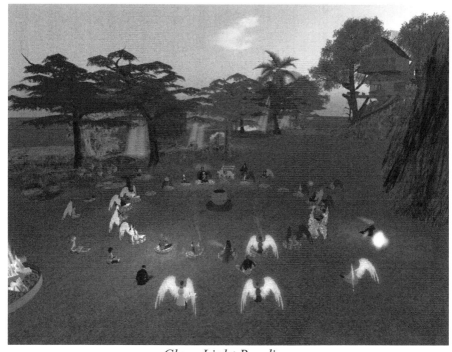

Clear Light Reading
Online Prosperity Path Ashram

DEH Notes August 4, 2017

Today was distinct from the other healing space-times so far.

A few minutes into the music, our healing space appeared before me and was functional throughout the event. There was no wormhole type event (as I might have hoped for).

I soon found myself quite some distance from the healing space and experiencing deities. Most were multi-armed, as that is what is needed to attend to the many facets of suffering everywhere. There was a circle of entities way "above" the Earth holding the larger space of the Earth-sphere.

There was a lot of holding space with certain postures held for quite some time, even though I don't normally do that sort of thing. Our original healing space was there, appearing as a small part of a much bigger arena/world.

The Ho'oponopono prayer came to mind early on and I was thinking: this is not the time to think about that, when it was made clear that, duh, this is part of the message for today.

There were two specific healing events.

At some point there was undifferentiated light-space. It was quite extraordinary. After about 25 minutes, perceptions normalized and it felt that other space had lasted forever.

I find it interesting how difficult it is for me to recall, even on the same day, what happened or how it was.

Relaxation, intention, openness, willingness for change are all ingredients of accessing the healing space – a space to recharge, reconfigure, transform. I am looking forward to next week and hope you will join.

Here is the story about the prayer I mentioned.

Hoʻoponopono prayer – a test of your practice

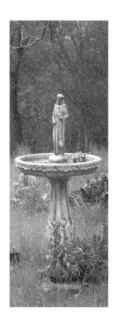

During the course of my work with animals in recent years, and expanding to plants, and on the basis of all the other things I had learned in my life, I had come to a place where it seemed to not make sense to have to kill anything to sustain my body. Around that time, I came across the description of sun-gazing, and BOOM, I started that week. I very quickly realized that I would never be able to complete this if certain emotional and mental states persisted – never mind how "right" I felt. This is when I remembered the modern **Hoʻoponopono** (ho-o-pono-pono) prayer, it's origin being an ancient Hawaiian practice.

When you do some googling, you will eventually find the story about the psychiatrist and the modern form of this practice/prayer and what happened to the psych ward full of crazy people. When you read the story – and I take it as true – you will be floored.

I had dabbled in using the prayer way back sometime, but the level of urgency and necessity, the relentless burning to BE, to walk this earth in a way to not cause any unnecessary harm to any sentient creature, and my love for animals and plants led me to face it for real. The thing about this prayer is: YOU are ultimately responsible – not just for your personal individual actions, but all of it. The adaptation of the practice is this prayer, four little phrases – to be said in any order – keeping the person or group of people you need to make things right within your mind:

I love you.

I am sorry.

Please forgive me.

Thank you.

Seeing all others as part of my own Self is what enabled me to do it with someone whose actions had caused me great pain. It does not make the actions right, but that is, frankly, irrelevant in this process. It is about YOUR inner state, and knowing that unless it changes, nothing in the outer will change. I should say that it took mere days for the effect to manifest. It is still a process, yes, but a big obstacle has been left behind. I don't think it will turn me into a very patient person anytime soon... but I am liking this effect of the prayer.

I have, since then, on occasion, put groups of people there who do those abominable things to animals, plants and the environment that is killing our very mother – Earth – who, like the sun, is also a Being, manifestation of consciousness.

I do work with non-physical guides, too, but this prayer, and to be able to say it for real – feeling it in your heart – is a test of your spiritual practice.

When I first started it, I kept wanting to say: "I forgive you." But no – it goes: "Forgive me." Even when you feel like YOU have been wronged. I know it makes no sense and you won't ever know that it does unless you try and when you discover why, that is another step on your path.

Much love to you.

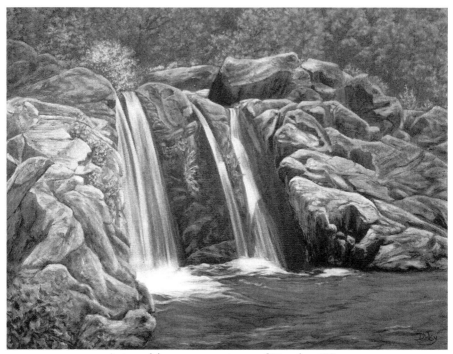

Art and image courtesy of Denise Wey

"The ultimate metaphysical secret, if we dare state it so simply, is that there are no boundaries in the universe. Boundaries are illusions, products not of reality but of the way we map and edit reality. And while it is fine to map out the territory, it is fatal to confuse the two."

~ Ken Wilber,
No Boundary: Eastern and Western Approaches to Personal Growth

DEH Notes August 11, 2017

Our healing space was there and very, very busy, surrounded in inter-penetrated by a larger energy, the kind that a couple of weeks ago seemed to be on the "other side" of the wormhole. The spaces are no longer appearing separate, but are actually occupying the same "space".

Today, there was one specific healing, but it took the form of not working on the actual body part, but only touching points on the head, synchronizing activity/waves/vibrations to induce a state of relaxation.

Several tuning-ins – as I am calling making connections with other beings.

Sometime halfway through the music, a huge love-space opened up. Not sure if anyone else could feel that. Visioning, imagining things and happenings while in that space – have creative manifesting effects in your life.

Later on, I kept getting this message to use a different music, even the name of the CD. So hm… "I" am not a fan of that, I admit resistance to it, but, I will get that music this week and we'll see how that goes next time.

Finally, been sitting here for a bit trying to remember… here is the message: Trust your body.

For that to start, tune into your body. How? What does that actually mean? You can start by paying attention to what actually happens in the body – feeling, sensations, aches and pains.

Pick a time when you are naturally quiet and not distracted and simply notice, letting your attention go to various parts of your body. Just notice what is there. You can also set yourself up to pay attention whenever in your daily life you remember this. Have a blessed week.

"...Because, you see, the alarming fact is that any realization of depth carries a terrible burden: those who are allowed to see are simultaneously saddled with the obligation to communicate that vision in no uncertain terms: that is the bargain. You were allowed to see the truth under the agreement that you would communicate it to others (that is the ultimate meaning of the bodhisattva vow). And therefore, if you have seen, you simply must speak out. Speak out with compassion, or speak out with angry wisdom, or speak out with skillful means, but speak out you must. And this is truly a terrible burden, a horrible burden, because in any case there is no room for timidity. The fact that you might be wrong is simply no excuse: You might be right in your communication, and you might be wrong, but that doesn't matter..."

~ Ken Wilber,

One Taste

DEH Notes from August 18, 2017

Today we used a different music as guided by a message from last week's healing event. Our healing space showed up fast and higher energy beings were working throughout. I did a few direct works, including opening a second chakra and then first chakra, then completing a general balancing. This was followed by another healing with a general balancing and working in the area of the third chakra. Both times this: you need to replace the habits with new ones.

The music today definitely caused a different space/vibration. While I did not resist it, the other music seems to be more conducive to a certain type of healing work and space. However, one thing was pretty remarkable and reminded me of an exercise during the LRS training – at some point each sound became a universe, seemed to stretch all the way to infinity.

At some point, there was that space of nothingness, lasting only a very short time for me, but come to think of it, I am not sure how I can keep standing up when the body seems to have disappeared.

I am grateful for this opportunity of serving in this way, of co-creating this space while at the same time holding it. We will use various sounds from now on as guided. For those who participated previously, I am interested in how you experienced the space this week, knowing that all the other times the music was the same divine harp music to support us.

Looking forward to our continued exploration into healing and transformation.

Much Love to you.

Christiane

"When you are inspired by some great purpose... dormant forces, faculties, and talents become alive, and you discover yourself to be a greater person by far than you ever dreamed yourself to be."

~ Pantajali

DEH Notes from September 1, 2017

Today it took a few moments longer to "see" our healing place, and when it came into view, it looked as if it had not been used for a while and most of the vegetation was dry and stunted. There were people there, but they were just there, having no clue about this being a place of healing or higher teaching. One family was sitting on some blankets close to the area that ended up being a portal last week.

I looked at the area and the wider view and there seemed to be less beings than in any other times, and generally, no one had much of an idea or intention about healing or a higher life.

I looked for the assembled group of our event and sure enough, the group was in a different plane located more to the left, a luscious healing space.

As I stood there overlooking the old healing space, I wondered if anyone there needed or wanted to connect. There was one. A child of about 3 or 4, dark skinned with an afro hairstyle. He saw me, telepathically asking, are you real, I answered and he wanted to touch, which he did, I told him he could lie on that special place on the ground and he did, falling through, but I was there were we were both floating in space. He was not afraid. Soon thereafter his mother told him to get back and then almost yanked him as they moved away, he looking back over his shoulder. I told him he can do this again.

There were three separate and specific healings after this.

There were a couple of messages, but I don't remember them. I'll add them if it comes back to me.

At some point our group's luscious place expanded to cover almost all the old healing area and, as if dripping energetically, beautiful energy and space came down until both places merged. The resulting space was not of this world, the being there were very integrated and highly evolved. Beautiful space/place to be.

There were a couple of other happening which I can't quite remember now. We reached a particular high space, but not as sustained as the last few times. The healing happened on a different vibrational level.

It was a very interesting event for me. I never know what will present itself when I stand there waiting in the beginning.

"Out beyond ideas of wrongdoing and right-doing, there is a field.

I'll meet you there."

~ Rumi

DEH Notes from September 8, 2017

Today, in the introduction, safety of the cells were a theme. Despite the ongoing fury the Earth is exhibiting, if you were at this healing, you are safe enough to go to a place to feel safe. It is sometimes necessary for your mind to understand that cells cannot grow and evolve when they are in protection mode. That is the current observed scientific finding. Threat makes cells, and organisms, develop and exhibit protective mechanisms, safety and nourishment makes them grow. For the human, Love is the most important ingredient for growth and development.

After a brief letting go of the outside world, all things in the past and plans for the future, we invited our higher self, the healing angels, Christ energy, higher vibrational forces, helpers and guides to aid in our transformation, for the benefit of all.

Once the music started, it took a few moments before the vision clarified to perceive anything on that level. What was before me was the healing square (a pretty large natural area surrounded by larger tress and bushes, as we have been at since the beginning). However, the space looked as it it had been deserted for a while, not even the transients were there anymore. It all looked pretty dry and the trees around the border were pretty dry, too. At the same time though, in the left front part of the healing space was a new, very lush green area with some healthy vibrant bushy trees and other vegetation. A couple of kids playfully peeked out from the area. It kinda looked like an oasis. Many a spring had opened up?

I did one healing which was mostly relational mother-daughter cord clearing. The mother shed "stuff" to come to a different place in herself, become much bigger. Another second healing is best described as core star activation.

Then I looked at that lush area again and went inside, and there was nothing, as in no bubbly spring or anything, well, almost nothing. Unlike the vast endless nothingness spaces visited in several of the other healing events, this one was very dark, but felt soft and contained. Being in it, there was gravity but no touching any ground, even standing up. It was quiet except for the music. It felt very, very… hm, safe in there actually. It was a very sweet space, and the cells really, really liked it. I could feel a whole section of my own cells come online, so to speak. There was a current of joy and curiosity and a willingness to move. Several of us were in that space dark space for some time.

Relaxation was possible and happened. Breathing was happening in a different way.

Oi, I know I am forgetting some things here.

This space felt more like an incarnational space to me, very different from the nothing vast spaces.

I am not sure there was an actual message today except I will share this realization: Safety for your cells to thrive is something you might have to create for them if that is not something they carry in their cellular memory.

All mothers: you cannot hold your infants too much. This letting them cry stuff is not the way to go. Get the support you need for yourself to be able to function, and get those newly arrived bundles held. The letting them have their own explorations on their own is for much later. In the process of incarnation, some things just work better than others.

Wishing you all abundance, joy and energy. May your healing journey continue.

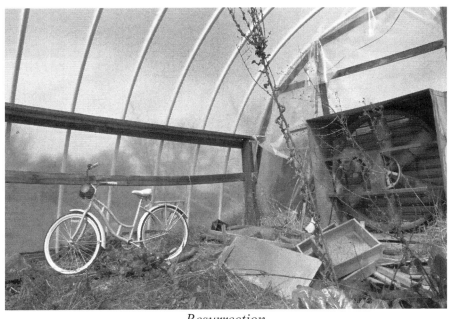

Resurrection
Image courtesy of Kathleen Dreier

Wherever you land, play there.

"You can't take control of your life by controlling your life."

~ E.J. Gold

"Don't be an end user."

~ E.J. Gold

DEH – Notes from September 15, 2017

Introduction and a bit of relaxation, together, with knowing that during the time of the healing, we can feel safe.

In the very beginning, before the healing space appeared before my eyes, there was a download, as I call it, visions of things I need to do as the next step. Lots of energy with it, though I am standing very still.

The healing space opened to view and I noticed how very parched the land looked. Even the area that looked like an oasis last time was struggling to stay green. There were no people or other organic beings when we started.

Then some showed up, healings were done, especially mother lineage past generation, but also body ailments that needed energy.

Then, there appeared a sea of beings, people in trouble. There was no way I could get through them, so I invoked massive amounts of healing energy from the higher realms to rain down on them and clear and cleanse.

There was a large group in the healing space and after energy infusion and cleansing, they were then given seeds, not by me, I just saw each and every one get a seed. To me, of course, they looked like plant seeds... but I know that for the most part they were seeds of ideas, next steps, something that is for those individuals to do, to continue or explore on this journey. My sense was that they were all relatively tiny steps, but this could be made up as it is just too particular for each one there... am writing this down to post it soon, so it can be read so you might more easily remember the thing that was YOUR seed.

Ask yourself if you were given something that is your seed, the seed for you to grow. And no, you don't know what it will look like once it develops.

Those entities (remember, the "people" appear to be as energy light beings) were then leaving, almost dismissed, and a whole new group showed up. The main characteristic of those was that they all seemed distracted. It is not that there is anything to do there, it was an internal disposition to be distracted. So, they were given (it appeared, I didn't "do" it) something to focus on. That something showed up as something large above the healing Plaza. It was in the shape almost like that of a candle flame, only it had no similarity in light to that of a candle. Pretty soon the entire group was focused and then, strings came out from that flame to connect with all the participants. Eventually everyone there, together, approached the central flame… and was eventually absorbed by it, after which the flame expanded enormously and then dissolved and all this energetic rain happened. Next thing I saw was the healing place transformed into a lush plaza with a gentle feel to it. There was a spring (never saw it there before) slightly to the right and slightly past the middle from where I stand. Beings came to get some water from it for sustenance then left, some briefly connecting with each other. They moved mindfully, but they did not come for healing per se.

I decided to go out into the field myself. It was so inviting. Once I reached about the middle of the space, I turned around… and saw myself still standing there at the edge. You would not recognize me, as it was not in the physical plane. Some interesting events happened there and later I looked back into the direction that is usually behind my back. It was a beautiful landscape, albeit did not have the feel of the healing space. Felt much more ordinary.

Beings kept coming and going to get water from the spring in the Healing Square. Those who came at that time were not there for healing, but nourishment.

Message: Drink from the fountain of the Inner Sanctum.

My reminder for you: What was your seed?

May all be blessed

Much Love to you

Christiane

158

The book I am writing is nearing completion and this was the last Distance Energy Healing event write-up to be included. As long as I am able, the Distance Energy Healing hour will continue on GorebaggTV. You are invited to be there. Let us heal together.

https://livestream.com/gorebaggtv/DistanceEnergyHealing

Notes of the healing hour will be posted online and be available for 1 week on this website: https://distance-energy-healing-with-dok.com/

I am also sending reminders through Facebook and will be posting on my new website: **https://let-the-healing-begin.com**

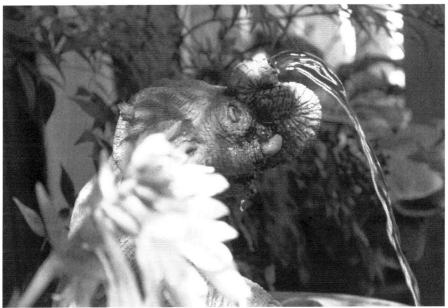

Froggy by the Fountain

As the Energy Healing events were taking place, it became clear that they are part of a process, and the form, and possibly purpose, will evolve. One thing that became obvious is that one of the functions of them is the maintenance, recharging and re-balancing of our energy bodies and a conscious re-alignment with the highest vibration possible in our lives. So much is going on in the world and our personal spheres. It impacts us. This healing opportunity for self care, relaxation together, recharging, realigning, and touching home is very welcome indeed. Thank you for participating.

Attitude is the Key!

All phenomena is illusion,
neither attracted not repelled,
not making any sudden moves,
my habits will carry me through.

~ E.J. Gold

From the American Book of the Dead

On the Shoulders Of Those Before Us

In various paths and schools, I have encountered the following thought/idea: One generation builds upon the successes and developments of the previous one, and as much as we are standing on the shoulders and work of those before us, so will the ones who follow our generation build on what those before them have accomplished.

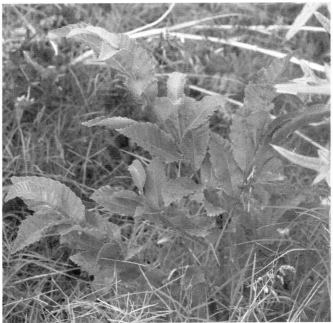

Baby chestnut tree, which I likely will never see fully mature.

Someday, someone might get lucky and be grateful for all the nuts.

Tom Brown Jr., The Tracker, said something similar, in that each class of the same name, he was teaching at a higher level. The same for the BBSH – each year the students would come in at a higher level.

The point is this: We learn, we take things as a given that the generation or two before us never even heard of. Even in my life as I look back on growing up, there was no word in school about quantum physics and its potential implications, no word about epigenetics, the nature of reality, or that maybe we are living in a simulation, no word on parallel universes, meditation or yoga. There was no internet. Yet, these days, there is much less rigidity and way more fluidity in considering the nature of things. Medically too, as I recall being taught that after the age of 2, the brain really does not develop much in the sense of forming new cells. These days we know how many days or weeks or months or years it takes for our organs to be 100% replaced. There is flexibility, plasticity, new learning and forging new pathways and neuro-circuitry. Genes are being switched off and on depending on our environment and experiences. What we eat influences our gut bacteria and they in turn can affect our mood through their metabolism.

The mindset that things are fixed can no longer be held as true, though, if you really insist on it, it will be true for you. The mindset that through learning, growing and practicing, you can change yourself is an important one to cultivate in healing. If you change the programming of your unconscious, you can change your life very fast.

The point I was getting at on this chapter is this: The people who came from a background of a particular density and conditioning have had to work in a certain way to extricate themselves from that morass, that confinement, that level of density, creating an energetic avenue, a blue-print, forging a path that then makes it easier for others to walk. Overall, each generation in the past 60 some years or so has had a higher degree of freedom and this is reflected in healing also. Have you noticed some kids these days are beyond amazing?

I come from a certain background and did a certain type of healing/consciousness work, as did scores of others. Many these days will not have to do that particular work and can build on a world that starts at a different baseline and can take humankind, and healing, further. Frankly, the faster the better, seeing the state of the planet.

Going deep, working with frequencies and direct transformation, i.e. what used to be called miracles, may soon be the cutting edge of health and healing. Working with clear intention and imagination is going to become much more important. Concentration and trust in the process of self-healing will be considered a given. Conscious alignment to a healthy blueprint with appropriate actions for compassionate self care will be commonplace. All this requires a much more integrated way of being than was the case for many of my own contemporaries. Meanwhile, keep grounding (connecting with the earth), be keenly aware of your thoughts and emotions, develop a mindset that allows for change to happen and keep at it, hang in there, don't give up if the miracle won't happen right away. Sometimes the miracle happens after a lot of hard work. Trust the process of life and Being itself. Invite and allow everything into your life that is for your highest good and for the benefit of all sentient beings everywhere and the benefit of the Absolute.

May this book have helped open a doorway for you with a vista of a better way of living for all, a view of a world and beingness which is new and full of potential, aligned with the highest good and beauty. The stepping through that doorway is something only you can do. It is something you need to be willing to do, to say yes to growth, change, transformation, and becoming whole. Step through the doorway to the next level, YOUR next level, no matter where you are at, no matter what your personal and cultural background may be. There still is the next step to take on your journey. Then you can take another step if it is needed for becoming more whole and integrated, if that is what you wish to do. I just think there will be another step, another level of where humans can go for a very, very long time. Just so you know, you will not have to give up your religion when you grow. You'll discover that too.

Me? I am just this one offering these online Distance Healing events and writing this book, due to something I named "the call", knowing that I am being part of a much larger whole, a tiny cog in the wheel of something super-big and eternal, a temporary expression of the "One". May I be a useful tool.

I sincerely hope you will join us for our healing hour on Fridays, giving yourself the gift of time for relaxation, self-care and healing. Once may be enough for whatever readjustment is needed to make your life more liveable, one time participating may be enough to start you looking around for the kind of help you need, or, you might participate often for repeated experiences of higher states of being, which eventually will add up toward the direction of your overall development and transformation. Maybe you will come as a practice and treasured time as often as you can, developing compassion for yourself, and, with that, for others. There is Love there waiting for you.

I feel grateful for all those who forged ahead and worked tirelessly for the benefit of all, and much gratitude for those of us who are working to pave the way for the next generation. Have you noticed some of the amazing young kids these day? I encourage you to call forth the next step, giant leap or tiny pitter-patter step, in your healing process.

I keep thinking of more things I wanted to let you know just in case those are the words that do it for you or transmit something I don't actually have words for. Hang in there! Find the funny side of things. Humor will get you through really, really difficult times. Learn to trust your intuition and allow curiosity and a sense of adventure at the doorstep into a new phase of life and being. May you walk with ease and grace – and don't forget to laugh often.

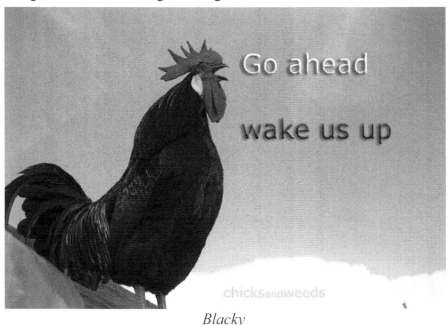

Blacky

Before I forget, in case you did not know: Dogs are heart energy beings – there is real and unconditional love expressed through them, their eyes, faces and bodies, that is easy to perceive and connect with. If you ever attempted to meet that, you know. They make openness and loving easily accessible to anyone in our culture, as they are living with us. They can do wonders for autistic children or people with PTSD and a lot of the rest of us.

This coming to center you might hear about, how is that done? It is sitting somewhere and slowing down, letting go of what your were thinking and doing or planning, letting it all go and connecting to your breath, your self, noticing your body, allowing thoughts but not hanging on to them, breathing into your belly, softly inviting love or peace, just being with any feelings, just being present.

You can invite help, higher energies, make a choice of what is important to you – loving from your heart, being true to yourself. It sets the tone for your way of being. If this resonates, you might like the Centering Prayer offered through the Christian Mystical tradition.

For those interested in states and stages, here is a quote from one of Ken Wilber's books:

"The difference between supermind and Big Mind (if we take Big Mind to mean the state experience of nondual Suchness, or turiyatita) is that Big Mind can be experienced or recognized at virtually any lower level or rung. Magic to Integral. In fact, one can be at, say, the Pluralistic stage, and experience several core characteristics of the entire sequence of state-stages (gross to subtle to causal to Witnessing to Nondual), although, of course, the entire sequence, including nondual Suchness, will be interpreted in Pluralistic terms. This is unfortunate in many ways – interpreting Dharma in merely Pluralistic terms (or Mythic terms, or Rational, and so on) – because it is so ultimately reductionistic; but it happens all the time, given the relative independence of states and structures at 1st and 2nd tier.

"Supermind, on the other hand, as a basic structure-rung

(conjoined with nondual Suchness) can only be experienced once all the previous junior levels have emerged and developed, and as in all structure development, stages cannot be skipped. Therefore, unlike Big Mind, supermind can only be experienced after all 1st-, 2nd-, and 3rd-tier junior stages have been passed through. While, as Genpo Roshi has abundantly demonstrated, Big Mind state experience is available to virtually anybody at almost any age (and will be interpreted according to the View of their current stage), supermind is an extremely rare recognition. Supermind, as the highest structure-rung to date, has access to all previous structures, all the way back to Archaic – and the Archaic itself, of course, has transcended and included, and now embraces, every major structural evolution going all the way back to the Big Bang. (A human being literally enfolds and embraces all the major transformative unfoldings of the entire Kosmic history – strings to quarks to subatomic particles to atoms to molecules to cells, all the way through the Tree of Life up to its latest evolutionary emergent, the triune brain, the most complex structure in the known natural world.) Supermind, in any given individual, is experienced as a type of 'omniscience' – the supermind, since it transcends and includes all of the previous structure-rungs, and inherently is conjoined with the highest nondual Suchness state, has a full and complete knowledge of all of the potentials in that person. It literally 'knows all,' at least for the individual."

~ Ken Wilber

The Fourth Turning: Imagining the Evolution of an Integral Buddhism

Facebook Post August 2017

Regarding the Distance Energy Healing event on GorebaggTV every week.

This is probably my longest post ever.

"Today, while stretching and relaxing prior to exercising, this thought occurred to me (in a more concrete way than before): To post this on Facebook with the "world icon" – opening it to the public.
A few weeks into the Distance Energy Healing live online, it has become clear to me how much I love doing them. I love the spaces accessed and I love that it has been beneficial for a number of people.

It is meant to reach a lot of you out there. All kinds of people, and decidedly not limited or geared to those with money, but anyone out there who feels things needs to change, things in their own life, things in themselves, anyone who is ready for accepting responsibility to move on, move up, grow up, anyone who wants to no longer be stuck and needs inspiration and a little boost.

So I am putting this out there so that many, many people may take advantage of this opportunity to be at the Distance Energy Healing event. People who would not be able to get other kinds of help, but are ready to take charge of their health, well-being and life in a different way. Folks ready to experience taking the time for themselves and self-compassion, take the time to slow down, relax and let inspiration come for what is needed in their lives and what steps they can actually do.

I am seeing groups of people, mostly small, gathered in a room where there is a computer and folks sitting or lying down entering a healing and transformative space, or mothers, kids in school – or participating, with enough time before lunch for this opportunity for transformational self-care and intentional relaxing for the purpose of healing, becoming well, regaining health, when otherwise they might simply not have the means to. Single, elderly or other folks who don't fit the usual American stereotypes, not that we know what that exactly means these days, but you get the drift. Or high level executives totally in the rat race, always performing – being able to slow down in the privacy of their own home.

During this Distance Energy Healing, you don't get to "watch", unless you wish to look at the altar, but you participate, even if you appear to do nothing. It is different from watching YouTube videos or listening to talks or reading articles. You are actually participating in this simple activity, which does not require any knowledge of meditation or mindfulness technique, does not require special equipment (computers these days are no longer special, but yes, necessary for the audio aspect of this), without having to talk, but able to ask questions via live chat the next time.

Of course I would like to continue doing this for as long as I can, and of course, eventually, the space I am using will have to stay supported. And of course, continuing to create a little corner of paradise, as temporary as it all may be, would be wonderful. So I am not saying money is not important in that way. My motivation is this: To help people grow and heal and when that happens, the world becomes a better place, and when people do better, all the other sentient beings will do better, too.

In any case, the book I wrote/am writing is being edited and hopefully will be available soon, and business cards are being worked on.

Giving anyone and everyone an opportunity and help to heal and grow, seems like the way to go. This is what I can do at this time. And I am doing it. May you be inspired to do what you are here to do from the deepest level of your being. May this opportunity lead to your up-leveling to a new phase.

As someone here said: the Distance Energy Healing events are happening, until they don't.

When? Fridays at 10:30 a.m. PST, on

https://livestream.com/gorebaggtv

168

The live event will be in the upper left. If not, we are having technical difficulties, which any thunderstorm could cause. Just tune in, event is still happening".

Admittedly, sometimes I, my thoughts, go into the direction of how meager this offering is comparing it to those who appear to be capable of so much more. Why embarrass myself? I see how true it is on one hand, and also how it is a playing of an old tape that was never mine to begin with. It was not mine. My spirit is bright, very bright. But oh, that stuff that happened on the incarnation path.

The answer is clear, because I love. There is love for this manifestation, our Earth and all the life on it. And looking at what is happening everywhere, change towards health and healing needs to happen fast for the sake of all those beings here, and this is my contribution at this time. I feel pulled and obligated. I am simply just one expression of all that is.

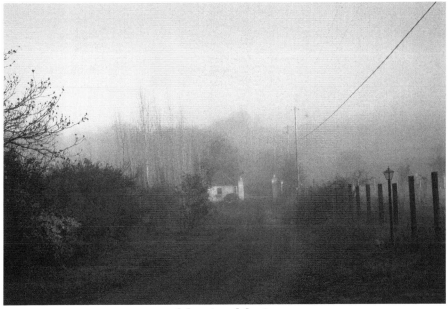

Morning Magic

The Speed of Light
Love is the speed of light.
The Absolute is love.
The Absolute is the speed of light.
The speed of light is stillness and silence.
The Absolute is stillness and silence.
Love is stillness and silence.
Where is stillness?
Between motion.
Where is silence?
Between sound.
Where is the Absolute?
Between motion and sound.
Silence between every sound.
Stillness between every motion.

~ E.J. Gold

Life in the Labyrinth

Practice, Habits and Exercises

There are some things on a journey of healing, transformation and awakening that are essential.

Here is one: you have to want it. Another: you have to be willing to discover and very likely change what you believe to be true.

Attitude is everything. E.J. Gold has gone this far: "Transformation is 100% attitudinal."

Change how you feel about something if you can't change the thing itself.

You have heard this: if you do what you have always done, you'll get what you always got.

If you want something different, you find ways to keep in focus, make it a priority, a goal, something worthwhile to you. Place it on your mental or physical list. If you can develop a passion for it, make it a top priority, develop a burning desire for it, all the better.

Imagine it happening, imagine and feel it being real, and love it.

To get through certain levels and transitions in your process, you also will need to free all the energy you can get. Do your shadow work.

Willingness to learn, to face your inner obstacles and asking for help if needed or changing your beliefs are all important aspects on this journey. But how do you even start?

Ok, you have set the healing intention, you are reading this book, you are invited to weekly online healings. Now what? Daily practice can help. In the following pages, I'll give you some ideas.

But why practice? Because such daily practice is, over time, transformational. It changes you. Over time, daily practice changes you and your life. Daily practice builds a certain type of inner will, respect for self, confidence, leads to expertise, transformation and healing. Deliberate daily practice changes your life, it helps you grow. You can be a good and successful person without daily practice, but there are things that you don't develop without it.

Developing a daily practice is worth it. Meditation and centering practices are good. E.J. Gold often recommends guitar, flute, doing jewelry or art practice, 5 minutes a day, but do it daily. Sounds easy enough – try it.

There are folks out there who offer all kinds of help with various programs you can follow. There is no point to keep talking about it, practice is something you need to do and personally experience.

First a clarification, in case of it being a question: a practice is not anything you already do for work, school, household maintenance or activities related to child raising or hobbies.

Practice is something extra, deliberate. I will give you a few examples that do not require money. Lack of money/funds is no excuse not to pick up a daily practice.

Here is my suggestion: try a practice you can do every day. Set yourself up for success. Pick a time that works for you. Set the duration at 1-5 minutes. For example, this easy one, as it requires only the use of a pencil and paper (and if you don't have that, use dirt/sand/mud and a stick): draw for five minutes a day. Draw anything. Yes, you are allowed to go online to find instructions, use DVDs or take a drawing class, but that is not the point: draw something every day. You will see how long five minutes can be, if you can even remember to do it. Therefore, pick a time and set yourself reminders that work to keep it up. Have your tools ready and visible.

On a day you are totally feeling overwhelmed, you can modify it to, at the very least, pick up the pencil (stick) and connect with it and the practice, even it you don't draw anything that day.

Also, you might need to commit to one week at first, then maybe one month, then, longer, one year or more. It is like building up a muscle. I am trying to say, set yourself up for success by making it something doable for you.

You can get started today. You can start a daily practice today.

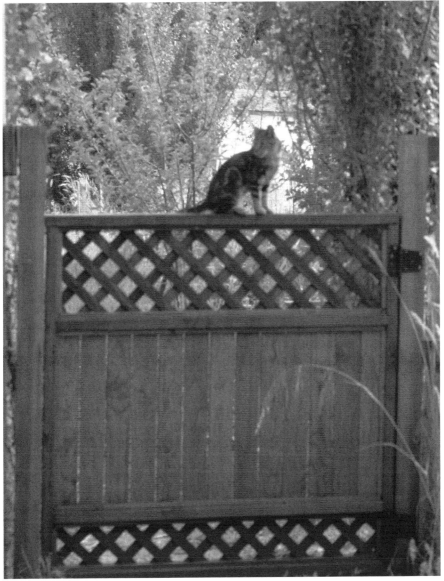

Up to You

No one can do it for you. It is a door you yourself have to step through.

More suggestions. If you have access to playdough, make something every day, as a practice.

Another good one is: get a cheap notebook and make a daily entry about your life. Could be a bullet point plan of things you want to do, or talk about something that happened, or decide you will talk about one feeling you had that day, every day.

Sit down somewhere once a day and imagine feeling happy, until you can feel it. Use any happy memories or future happy memories for this.

You can still do practice with your body. You can commit to do one stretch a day as a practice. You can expand this to planking, deliberate breathing, walking briskly, as a practice, and daily, 5 minutes, then 10 minutes, then 20 minutes, then 1 hour. Do it, see what happens.

Another free practice: be kind to someone every day. A person, an animal, a plant, as a practice. Not saying you need to limit being kind, but once a day, do it as a practice. You can go to the local animal shelter once a week and do your daily practice there, holding cats or puppies that day.

You can practice feeling grateful every day. Or see yourself very energetic. Feeling how that would be. Do it.

You can choose from lots of practices, just do them daily.

You can do one or more practices, like physical exercise, being kind, and draw, for a total of 15 minutes a day.

Here are some "easy" ones you can get started with if you are very new to any practice at all. I am reminding you that practice is not daily necessary chores, like taking kids to school, going to work, making coffee, feeding your animals. Practice is something you do for your development, to build something. You can, however, build a habit of cleaning your animal's bowls after each meal, or not let dishes build up in the sink, or make your bed before you leave the house.

You can commit to 5 minutes a day of guitar or flute practice, or singing, or drumming, or stretching, or lifting some weights, or drawing, carving, or embossing, or knitting, or sitting somewhere looking at a plant, or holding a rock, you know, things like that. Even just 1 minute, to keep the connection, but daily, do it as your daily practice. Check out practices that might work for you.

Every evening, you write down 10 things you feel grateful for. Pretty soon you could just keep writing and writing, but that is not the point, the point is to do a daily practice.

In the case of gratitude, it also changes the feeling state of your body and programs your autonomic nervous system for a different life.

You can pick a book and read at least one paragraph aloud daily. You can expand this to going to a nursing home once a week for your practice and read aloud there, maybe a poem, a beautiful story.

You can choose a question such as what is important right now and sit with it once a day.

Every day you can sit somewhere, take a deep breath and check in with your body, finding any area of discomfort, pain or uneasiness and tell your cells: I love you, I am here for you and I thank you – feel it.

You can do the same, every day, and find an area of the world that is hurting, and send it love, as much love as you are able to feel.

Whichever practice you choose, choose something you can be successful at, even if it means one minute, even if only for a week, renewing the commitment at that time. See if you can do a daily practice for 30 days.

There are other things you can do, such as remember upon waking up and before getting up to feel grateful for another day of opportunity for finding and living your life's purpose.

Are there other practices? Sure, some people are able to meditate or exercise daily for 1-3 hours. If you are just starting out, choose the 1-5 minutes one and do it every day.

After a while, you will realize the effects, you will make observations, notice things, be inspired to go deeper, or change the practice.

Remember, too, that eventually, or maybe even to start out, as the benefits are so needed, you want to include physical exercise as a practice, something for your mind like reading or writing and learning new things, be present with feelings, training attention, pick a mindfulness or contemplation practice.

In case you want to start with physical exercise: walk, stretch, do yoga poses, planking, lift weights (use filled water jugs if you must).

Eventually, a practice can become a habit. However, you don't really want it to become robotic.

You can, however, develop the habit to do practices.

Example of simple habit building: before eating or drinking anything on any given day, drink a glass of water each day.

Even if you become OCD about it, it is not a bad habit.

You will start to feel good about doing this thing for your body, and it will become easy.

Even if you take it a step further and make sure the water you drink does not contain chloride or fluoride, toxins from plastic or pharmaceutical residues, you still won't cause yourself harm. It will feel even better. The point here is: you can think of habits you want to develop that are beneficial to you and won't hurt even if they are automatic and that make you feel good to do.

You can ask yourself a simple question: if I do/say this, will it cause harm to anyone? Is it necessary that I say this, do this? What will be the effect of my saying/doing this on myself, or others? There are simple things, that don't cost money, you don't have to do it all day, just five minutes a day to start out.

If you are not in the habit of doing a daily practice, you might forget. Think of something to remind yourself.

There is no substitute for practice, there is not getting away from doing your part, your work. There is no quick fix done to you by a drug or the touch of a master. Those may at times lead to a high spiritual experience, but without the work, without doing your part, you'll be right back where you started very soon. And for transformation, practice is essential.

But we are back to the beginning: do you want healing, do you want a different life, do you want awakening?

Then YES.

Generally, habits can be replaced by other habits, but if you just stop a habit, something will fill the vacuum, usually the old habit.

There are attention and presence exercises you can do while doing your everyday activities. You will find the book: "Every Day a Holy Day" inspiring. Here is an example, paraphrased. While you are brushing your teeth: "Look into the mirror, take a moment and imagine the one you are seeing in the mirror is real, and you are the reflection."

If you like to play games, you can do exercises, called recipes in the book, while playing the game. "The Any Game Cookbook" is cool. Great if you play games with your kids or friends and I recommend: If you plan to do the recipes while playing a game, choose an easy game, like Shoots and Ladders, to start with (speaking from experience). Some recipes you can do without anyone being the wiser, some involve all the players participating.

Here is one from: "The Any Game Cookbook", reprinted with permission, without the graphic.

Sitting Like A Stone

The instructions are simple; it's just the application that's not so easy.

Recipe: During the playing of *any game*, allow your body, from the waist down, to go still. That means nothing moves, no fidgeting, no squirming, no moving of any kind. Arms, head, and upper torso move as usual. But below the waist, it is as if you were made of stone.

One might think that after making the intention to be still like a stone, it would be possible to shift one's attention to game play and simply ignore what's below the waist. Not so.

It will require constant vigilance to keep the legs *stoned*. To accomplish this effectively, you will need to split your attention, keeping a small portion of attention fixed upon your petrified legs.

If this recipe is a bit too difficult for the full course of a game, you could get an egg timer and activate the exercise during the course of one full draining of the sand. By turning the timer, you could alternate three minutes on, three minutes off.

In any case, you will eventually want to master doing this for a full hour of game play. But, don't dream this will happen the first, second, or even twentieth time you try. **You'd think with all the practice we get as couch-potatoes that this would be a snap. Think again.**

Here is another one from the same book:

Molasses Atmosphere

Day in, day out, we are swimming in an ocean of air. Because the air in this ocean is relatively thin, we don't notice. The air moves out of the way of our arms and legs so rapidly that we don't notice any drag or resistance from the air itself.

If we tried running in water, we would see and feel the resistance of the liquid around our legs and arms.

Imagine if we tried moving through an ocean of molasses. That is exactly what this recipe presents.

Recipe) While playing any game, move through the atmosphere as if you are living in an ocean of molasses.

Watching a group of players using this recipe while gaming is not unlike viewing Tai Chi Backgammon

You can do simple things like the "Touch a Rock" exercise. This Zen Basics meditation and attention trainer is available for instant download at zenbasics.com. You can watch the free video to see how it is done too. This is something you can do as a beginner, with groups with kids, and high level zen masters.

Always remember gratitude. Feel it. It will change you and your life.

A potentially challenging exercise might be this one: before going to sleep at night, imagine this was your last day and tomorrow you will not wake up. Feel what comes up for you.

There is a number that represents the sunrises you have remaining. Facing death, preparing for death – it is tempting to write yet another chapter, one about death, facing death, embracing death and living with death, just because it is so important for living, but I won't, mostly because there are other people who have explored and explained it much better and deeper than I have. What I will do is share the Clear Light Prayer at the end and this question: "What do you want to do with the time you have left on this Earth in this body"?

Many blessings to you on your journey of healing and transformation.

May you heal from the inside out and do what you came here to do

Much Love to you.

"Practice any art, music, singing, dancing, acting, drawing, painting, sculpting, poetry, fiction, essays, reportage, no matter how well or badly, not to get money and fame, but to experience becoming, to find out what's inside you, to make your soul grow."

~ Kurt Vonnegut

"What is The Work?
Forget all the BS you ever heard about it being too mysterious to mention. It's merely the combined effort of all Awakened Beings toward the Perfection of All Beings Everywhere which will greatly alleviate the suffering of the Absolute.

With your help it can be done."

~ E.J. Gold

Confronting the Clear Light

Now I am experiencing the Clear Light of objective reality.

Nothing is happening, nothing ever has happened or ever will happen.

My present sense of self, the voyager, is in reality the void itself, having no qualities or characteristics.

I remember myself as the voyager, whose deepest nature is the Clear Light itself;

I am one; there is no other.

I am the voidness of the void, the eternal unborn, the uncreated, neither real nor unreal.

All that I have been conscious of is my own play of consciousness, a dance of light, the swirling patterns of light in infinite extension, endless endlessness, the Absolute beyond change, existence, reality.

I, the voyager, am inseparable from the Clear Light;

I cannot be born, die, exist, or change.

I know now that this is my true nature.

~ E.J. Gold
From the American Book of the Dead

To Join the Online Healing Events

Distance Energy Healing with Dok is an online event and requires access to the internet to follow it directly. If you cannot attend live, you can participate through the archives, or simply tune in.

Distance Energy Healing

online via gorebaggtv

go to

https://livestream.com/gorebaggtv/DistanceEnergyHealing

Distance Energy Work and Healing Space

with

Dok and Higher Vibrational Energy Beings

This event is online/distance only – not onsite or hands-on

Date: Fridays – starting with orientation on June 2, 2017.

Time: 10:30 a.m. – 11:30 a.m. Pacific

Times may change, please check on IDHHB.com or distance-energy-healing-with-dok.com

Anyone is welcome to be in the space.

To indicate your wish to receive energy work, type OCD into the chat or speak "yes" in the space where you are. We invoke and ask guides, angels, Christ, and higher energy beings for help. No energy work happens without the agreement of your higher self.

We hold the intention for healing.

It is a safe space. Your cells, your body and being can relax and let the energy do any necessary work.

What you can do to prepare for the times/space includes:

- Create a space where you can be either lying down or sitting comfortably. You can also move, or do something like art work.
- Maybe have a mat or blanket to lie down on, pillows for knees etc., a cover or throw in case you get cool.
- If you have a Super Beacon, sit with it for a few minutes beforehand.
- Have any meaningful images or altar objects set up in the space if you wish (This could be angelic, Mother Mary, gods and goddesses, spirit guides, teacher-images, gemstones, photos, amulets etc.).
- Smudge the room if you can and appropriate where you live.
- Invoke or call on your higher self or higher vibrational beings to aid or work on you.
- Cultivate an attitude or willingness for change and towards wholeness, a willingness to let go of old patterns.
- If possible, turn your phone on vibrate and leave it elsewhere.

The above mentioned measures are recommended, but not mandatory or necessary. You may add your own, or simply tune in.

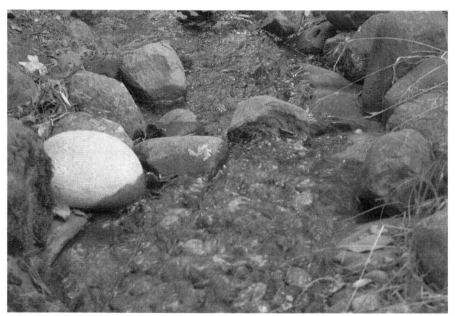

Happy Sounds

*"The secret of getting ahead
is getting started."*

~ Mark Twain

*"Between life's stimuli and our habitual
responses exists choice."*

~ *Ken Wilber*

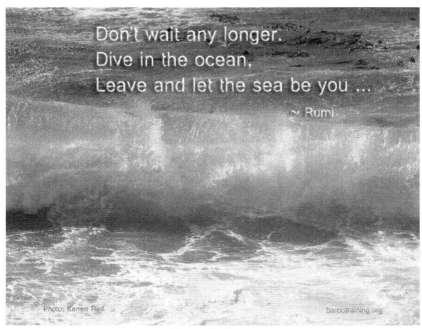

Pure Delight
Image Courtesy of Karen Reif

"Good for the body is the work of the body, good for the soul the work of the soul, and good for either the work of the other."

~ Henry David Thoreau

Acknowledgments

Most immediately I'd like to thank everyone who helped with the publication of this book, as well as IDHHB for making their broadcast system available.

To properly acknowledge everyone on my path would take a whole book in and of itself. Basically, everything and everyone. Still, some I will mention here: My birth family, especially my mom, dad, brother, sister and Oma, friends and teachers back in Germany. My love for nature is from way back then. There is my Brazilian family, adoptive families and friends and colleagues during my pediatric training and practice, various healing schools and modalities and the people who taught them. On this path, I have had many teachers and guides, but my first "real" "spiritual" teacher is someone I stumbled upon innocently when I attended the standard class of Tom Brown Jr, The Tracker, in 1990. I am not sure this would be happening if it were not for Tom Brown Jr and the Tracker School. Deep gratitude and respect for him and the teachings always. Some of my human helpers I would like to mention here are Karin and Ron Aarons (Temple of the Beloved) and Mukara Meredith (Matrixworks and Hakomi), Donovan and Susan Thesenga from the Pathwork. There were the folks at the Barbara Brennan School of Healing and the teachings and teacher there, the (then called) Waking Down in Mutuality path and teachers. Deep gratitude to E.J. Gold from the Institute for the Development of the Harmonious Human Being (IDHHB) for welcoming me home and developing all these tools for transformation and providing, most importantly, a work employment as well as a transformational cauldron. All along on my path, there were many influences via weekend workshops, countless books and later online events, classes and documentaries, with gratitude to all of you. There is the natural world and the Earth itself, not the least of which are the many chickens I accompanied in their life all the way through to the other side. And there was Skye, or, as I call her now, Bodhi-Skye, a German Shepherd Husky from the shelter, adopted in October 2010.

This is what I wrote about her back in 2011.

"I am essentially still speechless.

The adventure and voyage with her only lasted seven intense months. I am changed, and the course of my life has changed. And I am her – not separate – in the deepest heart of hearts. In essence, she will go with me to any manifest world. I had always known her and I always will. There is no time, (there) where I am her.

Little did I know it was to change my life, or – better said, change me, when I said YES to working with her. Even at the time I kept having the sense and visual of walking through a long tunnel with her. At some point towards the end there was an acute awareness of possible futures. I know I am different. There was a leveling up and integrating on a feeling level with the rest of "it". I am seeing people and things with a clarity that is mostly humbling and compassionate – and also seeing the extent of it all – with a peaceful silence, – and at the same time the energy to act.

She IS Art – sculpted and painted by nature and imbued with a big spirit by creation itself.

She IS Art – no point really trying to describe it – she is a delight to behold … beautiful, present, playful, regal, happy, alert, with such elegance in movement, with determination and focus, loyalty in doing her job – independent yet open to adjustment & contact – slowly giving her trust and turning into a love bug.

She raises your spirits with her magnificent presence just being who she is from her essence … a transmitter of divine vibration.

Maybe there are other dogs like this – maybe there is one such special dog for everyone that can have such an effect on someone. Maybe I was just ready to see, maybe she really is that special, maybe it was reawakening past life connection. Who knows …

186

I wish you could have seen her fly through the meadow, studying a situation, trying to play with a cow, or to teach Stormy how to play, or wag her tail.

May you be blessed with an encounter such as this, so when you hear someone say "it's just a dog" or "just a drum" or "just an animal" or "just a promise" or "just a weed" or "just a chicken" – you know that they "just don't understand"- not yet anyway. You've got to be open to the magic, willing to go through the portal into a different world, be amazed, accept what you find there, give it your full attention... allow your heart to be broken once again....humbled, still and awed – and be changed – ART... but really: LOVE."

She made me realize – that the grand being gets changed through us, and what we realize while alive through the deepest core of our being stays with us... and the Whole of what is, always.

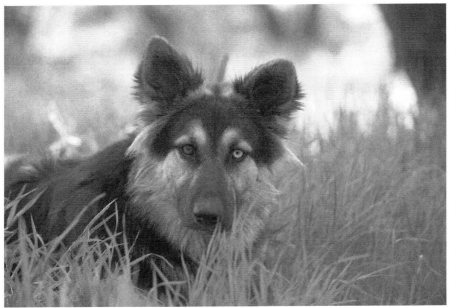

Bodhi-Skye – photo courtesy of Jim Rodney

"Until one has loved an animal, a part of one's soul remains unawakened."

~ Anatole France

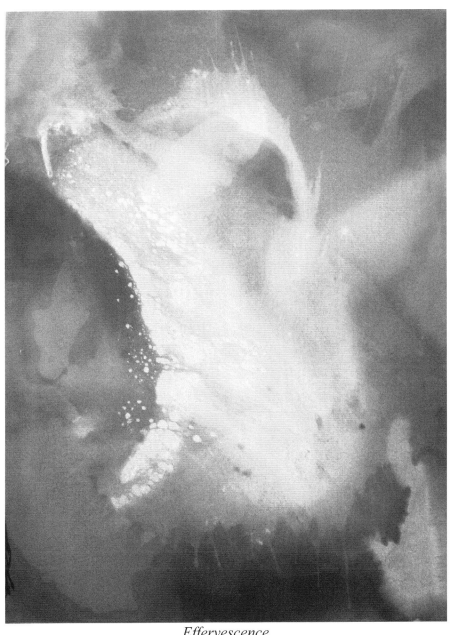

Effervescence

I renamed it to The Spirit Of Skye, that is what I see.

Art by Lil McGill

"Lying there on our deathbeds, we finally understand that the only thing left is our breath, God's love for us and our love for God, and anything we might have done to really work on and with the essential part of ourselves."

~ E.J. Gold

The Great Adventure

Abbreviations/Acronyms

ABD – American Book of the Dead

BBSH – Barbara Brennan School of Healing

BS – Bullshit

CBD - Cannabidiol

CME – Continued Medical Education

CQR – Crystal Quantum Radio

DEH – Distance Energy Healing

EFT – Emotional Freedom Technique

ER – Emergency Room

IDHHB – Institute for the Development of the Harmonious Human Being

LIRR – Long Island Rail Road

LRS – Labyrinth Readers Society

OCD – Open Channel DistanceEnergyHealing

PLS – Past/Parallel/Present Life Survey

PTSD – Post Traumatic Stress Disorder

PVA - Prosperity Virtual Ashram

"The understanding of 'evolutionary consciousness' is perhaps the most important thing lacking in spiritual practices today. Evolution means growth and development. This means that there are aspects of reality that have not yet arisen in our consciousness. But they will arise if we grow."

~ Ken Wilber

Recommended Reading

Tom Brown's Field Guide to Nature and Survival for Children - Tom Brown, Jr

Hands of Light - Barbara A. Brennan

Light Emerging - Barbara A. Brennan

Any Game Cookbook   Recipes for Spiritual Gaming - Claude Needham

Every Day a Holy Day - Barbara Haynes

Practical Work on Self - E.J. Gold

Ender' s Game - Orson Scott Card

Grace and Grit - Ken Wilber

The American Book of the Dead - E.J. Gold

Your Dog is your Mirror - Kevin Behan

Das geheime Leben der Bäume - Peter Wohlleben
(The Hidden Life of Trees)

You can find out more about Distance Energy Healing with Dok on this website:

let-the-healing-begin.com

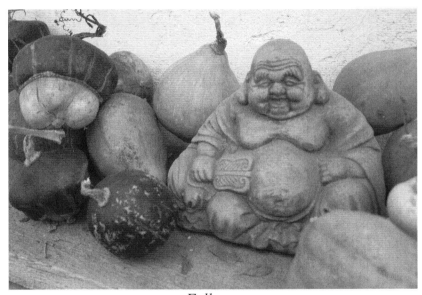

Fullness

"Let The Healing Begin"

by

Dr. med. Christiane Wolters, M.D.

For more information and updates

go to

let-the-healing-begin.com

distance-energy-healing-with-dok.com

IDHHB contact information:

IDHHB

PO Box 370

Nevada City, Ca, 95959

tel

1-800-869-0658

1-530-271-2239

http://idhhb.com

http://gatewaysbooksandtapes.com